Studies in Computational Intelligence

Volume 631

Series editor

Janusz Kacprzyk, Polish Academy of Sciences, Warsaw, Poland
e-mail: kacprzyk@ibspan.waw.pl

About this Series

The series "Studies in Computational Intelligence" (SCI) publishes new developments and advances in the various areas of computational intelligence—quickly and with a high quality. The intent is to cover the theory, applications, and design methods of computational intelligence, as embedded in the fields of engineering, computer science, physics and life sciences, as well as the methodologies behind them. The series contains monographs, lecture notes and edited volumes in computational intelligence spanning the areas of neural networks, connectionist systems, genetic algorithms, evolutionary computation, artificial intelligence, cellular automata, self-organizing systems, soft computing, fuzzy systems, and hybrid intelligent systems. Of particular value to both the contributors and the readership are the short publication timeframe and the worldwide distribution, which enable both wide and rapid dissemination of research output.

More information about this series at http://www.springer.com/series/7092

Robert Koprowski

Image Analysis for Ophthalmological Diagnosis

Image Processing of Corvis® ST Images
Using Matlab®

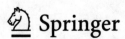

Springer

Robert Koprowski
Division of Biomedical Computer Science,
  Faculty of Computer Science
  and Materials Science
University of Silesia
Sosnowiec
Poland

Additional material to this book can be downloaded from http://extras.springer.com.

ISSN 1860-949X   ISSN 1860-9503   (electronic)
Studies in Computational Intelligence
ISBN 978-3-319-80595-5   ISBN 978-3-319-29546-6   (eBook)
DOI 10.1007/978-3-319-29546-6

This Springer imprint is published by SpringerNature
The registered company is Springer International Publishing AG Switzerland

Foreword

Numerical image processing is a rapidly growing interdisciplinary field of science that allows for quantitative analysis of processed images in order to extract certain characteristic physical properties and features of objects, contained in the analysed images of these objects. These properties can be encoded both in individual images and image sequences. One of the main areas of application of numerical image processing is biomedical research and diagnostics. It is impossible to enumerate all fields of biomedicine in which images and their sequences are recorded and then processed numerically. They range from computer tomography to phase micro-scopy methods.

In many cases, ophthalmological diagnosis and examination of the eye also use numerical image analysis. One such example is the Corvis® ST OCULUS, a non-contact tonometer for measuring intraocular pressure (IOP) and other corneal properties. The tonometer uses a very fast Scheimpflug camera, which records a video sequence of deforming cornea due to an air-puff from the device nozzle. Numerical analysis of images in a sequence allows for the quantitative description of the geometry changes of the deforming cornea. Such changes enable to measure IOP in the anterior chamber of the eye and other important corneal characteristics. It turns out, however, that the problem of measuring IOP is much broader and more complex than it is thought. The air-puff pressure from the nozzle causing rapid deformation of the cornea has to overcome not only the pressure in the eye but also the resistance of the cornea itself, resulting from its biomechanical properties. This constitutes one of the causes of inaccuracies in IOP measurements with the use of different types of tonometers. So far, the biomechanical properties of the cornea cannot be fairly accurately measured in vivo. This measurement, however, could be very useful in the advanced ophthalmic diagnosis and in increasing the accuracy of IOP measurement.

A more detailed analysis of the corneal deformation over time, based on the advanced numerical processing of images recorded by the Corvis tonometer, can contribute not only to increasing the accuracy of IOP measurement and, developing new methods of measuring the biomechanical properties of the cornea, but also to broadening our knowledge about the cornea and anterior chamber of the eye.

For this reason, the book fits perfectly into the mainstream of contemporary studies of the eye and may contribute to the development of modern diagnostic methods in ophthalmology. The image processing methods and algorithms described in the book can be applied in a number of other important studies and measurements which use image registration.

Wrocław   Henryk Kasprzak
October

Preface

Medical diagnostics has been supported by image analysis and processing for many years. Nowadays it is very difficult to imagine image diagnostics without the use of image analysis and processing tools. All types of devices such as optical tomography, ultrasound or X-ray equipment often have advanced possibilities of image manipulation and processing. These operations, performed directly in images, facilitate decision-making. These are mostly features of the images (both 2D and 3D) themselves. For example, the number and parameters of objects in the image or their distribution relative to the adopted coordinate system are analysed. This enables to calculate the progress of retinal detachment treatment, the degree of spinal curvature and the degree of colour reaction of cells in microscopic imaging, or diagnose Hashimoto's disease in ultrasound imaging. The methods for tracking the movements of individual objects or subsequent analysis of their trajectories are found equally often. For example, there is tracking of sperm trajectories necessary for the assessment of its mobility, tracking of insects needed to assess their behaviour or analysis of cell proliferation in microscopic imaging. In each of these cases the base are image analysis and processing methods profiled for a particular application. The need to profile them results from the nature of biological and medical images and, above all, high inter-individual variability of patients. On the other hand, the proposed methods should be versatile enough to work well in different medical centres for different types of patient populations. Maintaining the right balance between these two elements is generally implemented through an appropriate algorithm structure. The algorithm sensitivity to changes in parameters (e.g. the position of the patient relative to the imaging device) and algorithm features, such as fully automatic measurement and repeatability of the results, are important here as well. One such type of devices requiring a profiled algorithm for image analysis and processing is the Corvis® ST, OCULUS Optikgeräte GmbH, Germany (hereinafter abbreviated to Corvis). In this tonometer, using the proposed algorithm, it will be possible to measure parameters related to corneal deformation or the eyeball reaction over time.

This book is therefore suitable for both researchers who want to expand their knowledge on the use of image analysis and processing methods in the Corvis tonometer and students of computer science and bioengineering. The presented algorithms were implemented in MATLAB$^©$ (hereinafter abbreviated to Matlab) and tested in practice. Therefore, this book is also addressed to doctors, particularly ophthalmologists who by using the described methods can gain new and diagnostically important features of the cornea and eyeball. However, due to the considerable complexity of algorithms, a basic knowledge of Matlab is required from the reader.

The described algorithms have been presented in this monograph in the form of Matlab source code. The choice of Matlab results from its versatility in various fields of science. Owing to numerous toolboxes, it can be applied not only in image analysis and processing but also in economics, electronics or statistics. An extension of these known toolboxes is a group of algorithms presented in this monograph. They are also available in the form of m-files attached to this book. It should be emphasized here that the presented algorithms are only one of the possible solutions to a given problem and do not exhaust this very interesting subject.

The presented algorithms may also be used to solve other problems occurring in automatic biomedical image analysis. Some selected as well as all of the presented algorithms may also be applied, for example, in the analysis of X-ray and thermal images as well as images from CT where full automation and repeatable results are essential.

Acknowledgments

First of all, I would like to thank Prof. Henryk Kasprzak from the Wroclaw University of Technology, with whom I have always been happy to discuss topics related to eye metrology. These discussions resulted in several works mentioned in the list of references which inspired me to develop subsequent versions of the algorithm and to write this monograph. Close collaboration with Prof. Edward Wylegała and his team from the Railway Hospital in Katowice has allowed me to become familiar with the issues of corneal deformation in terms of clinical practice. As a result of this collaboration, several further papers were produced describing the possibility of using data analysis methods in clinical diagnosis. I express equally warm thanks to Dr Sven Reisdorf from Oculus for providing the sequence of images presented in this study and his consent to use it. I also thank my colleagues with whom I exchanged many insights and ideas related to tonometry: Dr. Renato Ambrósio Jr. from the Instituto de Olhos Renato Ambrósio, Brazil, and Dr. Lei Tian from the Department of Ophthalmology, Chinese PLA General Hospital, China.

In particular, I would like to thank Professor Zygmunt Wróbel from the Department of Biomedical Computer Systems, University of Silesia, Poland and Dr. Sławomir Wilczyński from the Silesian Medical Academy for a long-term cooperation and help.

Particularly warm thanks to my immediate family, especially my wife Agnieszka, for her daily help during writing this monograph.

I am also thankful to many others not mentioned here.

Contents

Symbols

m	Row
n	Column
i	Number of the image in a sequence
$L(m,n)$	Point of the matrix of the image L
M	Number of rows in a matrix
N	Number of columns in a matrix
I	Number of images in a sequence
q_w	Number of quantization levels
q	Number of edge portions
h	Filter mask
SE	Structural element
p_r	Threshold
δ_g	Measurement error
FP	False positive
FN	False negative
TP	True positive
TN	True negative
TPR	True positive rate
SPC	Specificity
ACC	Accuracy
d	Noise density
T	Time constant
$G(s)$	Transmittance

Chapter 1
Introduction

1.1 Purpose and Scope of the Monograph

The purpose of this monograph is to propose methods for analysing and processing of images from the Corvis tonometer. These methods should have the following specifications:

- fully automatic measurement—no operator intervention in the analysis process,
- reproducibility of results—the obtained results should be identical for the same sequence of images,
- resistance to inter-individual variability of patients—the algorithm should work well for various types of diseases of the eye or cornea and for different patient populations,
- availability of the full source code of the algorithm in Matlab.

The next chapters focus on the successive phases of analysis and processing of images from the Corvis tonometer. This first chapter presents the basic definitions used further in the monograph. The second chapter is devoted to the acquisition and pre-processing of images. Attention was also paid to such issues as image normalization or histogram equalization. The third chapter presents the main image processing and provides a detailed discussion of its subsequent stages and the used source code. In particular, it describes the known and (three) new methods of corneal edge detection. The third chapter ends with the comparison of the proposed new edge detection methods. The fourth chapter is devoted to additional measurements and analyses based on the detected corneal edge. These include measurements which provide some new information (data) related to the biomechanical characteristics of the cornea or the eyeball as well as the advanced stages of image analysis and processing, e.g. texture analysis of the cornea. The fifth chapter shows the properties of the proposed algorithm. In particular, it discusses the algorithm

© Springer International Publishing Switzerland 2016
R. Koprowski, *Image Analysis for Ophthalmological Diagnosis*,
Studies in Computational Intelligence 631, DOI 10.1007/978-3-319-29546-6_1

sensitivity to parameter changes and measurement errors. The last sixth chapter is the summary of the developed algorithm and obtained results. This chapter also presents the final version of the application designed for automatic measurement of the discussed parameters.

1.2   Material

The images were acquired from the Corvis ST (OCULUS Optikgeräte GmbH, Germany). Each of the 2D images had a resolution $M \times N = 200 \times 576$ pixels (16.5×15.7 µm/pixel). $I = 140$ 2D images were recorded for a single eye. The presented algorithm was tested for 50 image sequences—each sequence had 140 2D images. The sequence of (140) 2D images was directly related to the eye response to an air-puff generated by the Corvis tonometer. Each 2D image is recorded automatically in the Corvis tonometer using an Ultra-High-Speed Scheimpflug camera. This camera enables to acquire 140 such images in 32.11 ms, which means that the time interval of obtaining successive images is 231 µs. It should be emphasized here that for the purposes of this monograph, no studies, measurements or tests were performed on humans. The algorithms were tested on retrospective data. Image sequences, together with consent for publication, were provided by OCULUS. The images were obtained in accordance with the Declaration of Helsinki with free and informed consent of patients and were taken with the participation of a specialist. The selected tiny portions of the algorithm presented in this monograph were tested for a larger population of healthy subjects and ill patients (keratoconus and others) and described in detail in [1–3].

1.3   State of the Art

Corneal deformation includes an interdisciplinary range of three areas:

- computer science—image analysis discussed in this monograph,
- mechanics—an explanation of phenomena, mainly dynamic ones, occurring during corneal deformation and,
- ophthalmology—understanding the phenomena which accompany corneal deformation—such as the impact of the type of disease or the eyeball reaction.

The three above-mentioned areas have been described in literature to varying degrees. Now, in the years 2015–2016, there are intensive attempts to connect the mathematical model with the recorded data and the type of disease.

In the area of mechanics, there are numerous approaches to model the cornea using the finite element analysis or simple deformation analysis methods. These are mainly the works of Elsheikh [4, 5] on the influence of epithelium on corneal biomechanical properties, and the works of Roberts [6–14] on corneal vibration and the impact of pachymetry or patient's age on the results obtained. The doctoral thesis of Kling [15] was also devoted to this area, namely biomechanics. The works on the influence of selected diseases on biomechanical properties are equally interesting. These include the works of Brown [16], Dupps [17], Elisheikn [4, 5], Fontes [18], Hassan [19], Kotecha [10, 20] and many others [12, 21–27]. They concern in particular the problems of refraction and its links with biomechanics of the cornea.

In ophthalmology, the impact of intraocular pressure and keratoconus on corneal biomechanical parameters is mainly examined. These parameters are obtained directly from the Corvis tonometer when measuring intraocular pressure. The issues of this type are investigated by Wylegala [28], Ambrósio [18, 29], Lei [30], Lanza [31]. There are also publications in the field of ophthalmology and corneal deformation related to the impact of treatments such as LASEK (laser-assisted sub-epithelial keratectomy) [32], LASIK (laser-assisted in situ keratomileusis) [25], lenticule [33], corneal refractive surgery [19], primary open-angle glaucoma [34], penetrating keratoplasty [35] or visual field testing [36] on biomechanical properties. The analyses presented in the above works concern biomechanical parameters provided by the Corvis tonometer and their use in the classification of healthy subjects and patients having these diseases (e.g. keratoconus). The classification results obtained in all of these works are statistically significant.

The last area directly linked with the Corvis tonometer is image analysis. Currently, there are a few studies which allow for semi-automatic or fully automatic determination of corneal contours on a sequence of corneal deformation images. These are the works of Lei [37] and Koprowski [1–3, 38, 39]. They assess the possibility to detect the corneal contour on a sequence of images from Corvis. Moreover, the works [1, 3] discuss additional parameters obtainable from the proposed algorithm. The work [38] shows the impact of the extraocular muscles on the registered response to an air-puff from the tonometer. These works are dominated by classical methods of contour detection such as the Canny method or morphological gradient. The used filters are mostly median filters and the presented methods of morphological operations are mainly erosion, dilation as well as opening and closing operations formed on their basis. The presented methods, however, due to the limited volume of the said articles, only provide the block diagram of the algorithm without presenting the theoretical foundations necessary for its development and, in particular, its source code. This prevents wider use and testing these methods for other cases. This monograph systematises this knowledge and describes individual stages of creating applications for the analysis of images obtained from the Corvis tonometer. Additionally, the described new methods of image analysis allow for the acquisition of new biomechanical characteristics and assessment of their suitability in practice.

1.4 Basic Definitions

1.4.1 Coordinate System

Individual points in a 2D image were defined as a two-dimensional function $L(m, n)$ where m and n are the coordinates, and the amplitude is defined as the L value for a pair of coordinates (m, n). The function amplitude L is directly linked to the intensity function or the Luminance brightness function (the L symbol is derived from the first letter of the word) [1].

The L function is generally represented by a 2D matrix. Two coordinate systems associated with the matrix will be used: one related to geometric coordinates (Fig. 1.1) and the other one (used more often) related to the arrangement of rows and columns in the image matrices (Fig. 1.2).

The order of giving the individual dimensions of the matrix (Fig. 1.2) was adopted in accordance with the nomenclature used in Matlab, FreeMat, Scilab or Octave. The first dimension is the row, the second dimension is the column and then there are other dimensions, wherein the numbering of these dimensions starts with one instead of zero. This is common numbering used in most of the publications devoted to image analysis and processing (Fig. 1.2). Thus, the specified

Fig. 1.1 Image in the geometric coordinate system with *points* indicating brightness function domain pixels and *squares* representing detector sensors

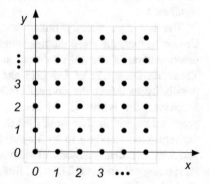

Fig. 1.2 Image in the screen coordinate system represented in the form of an array (m—row, n—column)

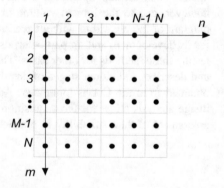

coordinate system enables to define resolution as a pair of values $M \times N$, where M is the number of rows of the image matrix and N is the number of columns, i.e.:

$$L(m,n) = \begin{Bmatrix} L(1,1) & L(1,2) & \cdots & L(1,N-1) & L(1,N) \\ L(2,1) & L(2,2) & \cdots & L(2,N-1) & L(2,N) \\ \vdots & \vdots & & \vdots & \vdots \\ L(M-1,1) & L(M-1,2) & \cdots & L(M-1,N-1) & L(M-1,N) \\ L(M,1) & L(M,2) & \cdots & L(M,N-1) & L(M,N) \end{Bmatrix}$$

(1.1)

The image function L was defined as:

$$L(m,n): C \times C \to C^+ \cup \{0\} \tag{1.2}$$

When the L function can take floating-point values, it can be written in the following way:

$$L(m,n): C \times C \to R^+ \cup \{0\} \tag{1.3}$$

The individual function values are determined: on the set of integers $(C^+ \cup \{0\}) \cap [0, q_w - 1]$, $q_w \in C$ of quantization levels (generally $q_w = 2^8 = 256$); or on the set of floating-point numbers, this is the range $[0, 1]$. Floating-point numbers are also written according to the nomenclature adopted in Matlab with dots as decimal separators. However, the individual elements (figures) are separated with a space or comma.

1.4.2   Contour and Edge

The contour in a monochrome 2D image is a line in the case of continuous structures or a group of pixels in the case of discrete structures. These are the points of the image function L, in the simplest case, with a constant brightness value. In the general case, they are directly linked with the object edges which are defined as physical, photometric and geometric points of the image function discontinuity. The edge is formed on the border of areas with different values of the image function L. The edge is the contour of the object. The most common and typical example of the edge including noise is shown in Fig. 1.3, where four cases are highlighted: (a) the ideal step profile, (b) the smoothed step profile, (c) the object with rising edges (d) the object with step edges.

Depending on the scale of consideration, the edges may also be classified as objects. This distinction is dependent on the definition of the object, and especially its minimum size.

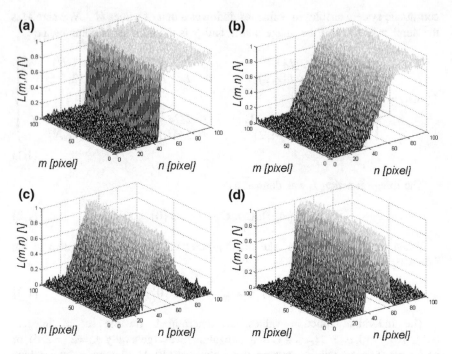

Fig. 1.3 Transverse profiles of the edges and objects in the image **a** the ideal step profile, **b** the smoothed step profile, **c** the object with rising edges **d** the object with step edges

1.4.3 Known Edge Detection Methods

According to the afore-mentioned definition of the edge, it seems that the easiest way to detect it is to use differentiation operations. They provide information about brightness changes of the input image. For the sample image $L(m, n)$ shown in Table 1.1, a profile of grey level changes $L(m^*, n)$ was formed, where m^* is a constant value and in this case $m^* = 50$ (see Fig. 1.3).

On this basis, it is possible to calculate:

$$\frac{\partial L(m, n)}{\partial n} = \lim_{\Delta n \to 0} \frac{L(m, n + \Delta n) - L(m, n)}{\Delta n} \tag{1.4}$$

In the discrete case, it can be assumed that Δn is equal to one pixel, i.e. $\Delta n = 1$, and then:

$$\frac{\partial L(m, n)}{\partial n} \hat{=} \Delta_n = L(m, n + 1) - L(m, n) \tag{1.5}$$

Table 1.1 Various stages of edge detection using information about the gradient

Symbol	Image/Graph
$L(m*, n)$	
$\frac{\partial(L(m*,n))}{\partial n}$	

Similarly for the image axis m, i.e.:

$$\frac{\partial L(m,n)}{\partial m} \hat{=} \Delta_m = L(m+1,n) - L(m,n) \tag{1.6}$$

The results of the differentiation operation for $m* = 50$ calculated according to the formula (1.5) are shown in the table below (Table 1.1). As is apparent from the results shown in Table 1.1, calculating the derivative in the designated direction (in this case along the m-axis) in accordance with the definition does not produce the desired results. The image $L(m, n)$ should be filtered out using any method, so that local changes in the pixel brightness will not affect the result. In this case, filtration is carried out through, for example, convolution of the image $L(m, n)$ with the mask $h(m_h, n_h)$, wherein the mask will be understood as the kernel, in this case, the Gauss transform, i.e.:

$$h(m_h, n_h) = \frac{1}{2 \cdot \pi \cdot \sigma^2} \exp\left(-\frac{m_h^2 + n_h^2}{2 \cdot \sigma^2}\right) \tag{1.7}$$

where σ is the standard deviation.

The filter mask has a resolution $M_h \times N_h = (2 \cdot m_w + 1) \times (2 \cdot m_w + 1)$ with the centre of the coordinate system located at the point (m_0, n_0). On this basis, the convolution was carried out according to the known equation:

$$L(m, n) * h(m_h, n_h) = \sum_{m_h=m_0-m_w}^{m_h=m_0+m_w} \sum_{n_h=n_0-n_w}^{n_h=n_0+n_w} L(m - m_h, n - n_h) \cdot h(m_h, n_h) \quad (1.8)$$

In the one-dimensional case, where $m =$ const. (hereinafter referred to as $m*$), using the first derivative of the function and convolution operation enables to create the edge detector. Then the location of the edge can be determined after performing an elementary binarization operation on the waveform $\partial(L(n) * h(n_h))/\partial n$—Table 1.2.

On the basis of the problem formulated above (and Table 1.2), in practice, Roberts masks are defined directly from the differentiation definition (1.4), Prewitt masks—using the Taylor series expansion of the function $L(m, n)$, and Sobel masks—taking into account the wheel proximity and Kirsch compass operator [40].

The second group of detectors is based on finding zero crossings of the second derivative of the function $L(m, n)$. Similarly to (1.5) and (1.6), in the discrete case and with the shift on the n-axis, it can be written as:

$$\frac{\partial^2 L(m, n)}{\partial n^2} \hat{=} \Delta_n \Delta_n = L(m, n+1) - 2 \cdot L(m, n) + L(m, n-1) \quad (1.9)$$

similarly for the image axis m, i.e.:

$$\frac{\partial^2 L(m, n)}{\partial m^2} \hat{=} \Delta_m \Delta_m = L(m+1, n) - 2 \cdot L(m, n) + L(m, n+1) \quad (1.10)$$

As in the case of the first derivative, detectors based on the second derivative are very sensitive to the slightest change in grey levels. For this reason, pre-filtration with the Gauss filter is performed, yielding the results presented in Table 1.3.

The equation from the theory of convolution was used in Table 1.3:

$$\frac{\partial^2}{\partial n^2}(L(n) * h(n_h)) = L(n) * \left(\frac{\partial^2}{\partial n_h^2} h(n_h)\right) \quad (1.11)$$

In the case of a two-dimensional function, the Laplace operator can be defined on this basis as:

$$\nabla^2 L(m, n) = \frac{\partial^2 L(m, n)}{\partial m^2} + \frac{\partial^2 L(m, n)}{\partial n^2} \quad (1.12)$$

The use of the Eqs. (1.11) and (1.12) in the Gauss transform (1.7) results in:

Table 1.2   Various stages of edge detection using the gradient and convolution with the Gaussian kernel

Value	Image/Graph
$L(m^*, n)$	
$h(n_h)$	
$L(n)*h(n_h)$	
$\frac{\partial(L(n)*h(n_h))}{\partial n}$	

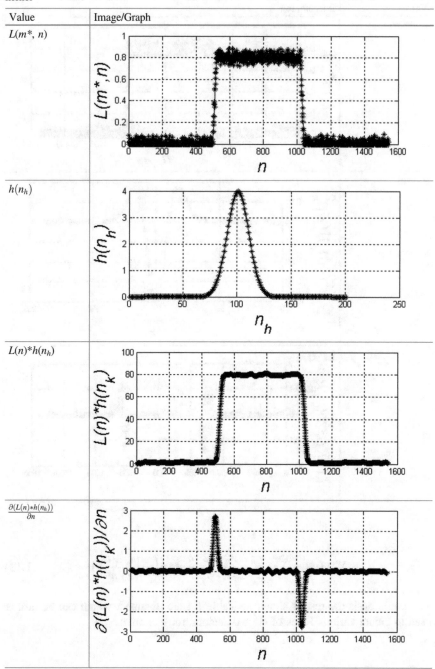

Table 1.3 Various stages of edge detection using the second derivative and the Gauss filter

Value	Image/graph
$L(m^*, n)$	
$\frac{\partial^2(h(n_h))}{\partial n_h^2}$	
$L(n) * \frac{\partial^2(h(n_h))}{\partial n_h^2}$	

$$\nabla^2 h(m_h, n_h) = \frac{m_h^2 + n_h^2 - 2 \cdot \sigma^2}{2 \cdot \pi \cdot \sigma^6} \exp\left(-\frac{m_h^2 + n_h^2}{2 \cdot \sigma^2}\right) \qquad (1.13)$$

On this basis the results shown in Table 1.4 are obtained, which can be further used to create various types of edge detectors, for example:

Table 1.4 Gauss mask, its first derivative after n_h, m_h and Laplacian

Value	Graph
$h(m_h, n_h)$	
$\frac{\partial h(m_h, n_h)}{\partial n_h}$	
$\nabla^2 h(m_h, n_h)$	

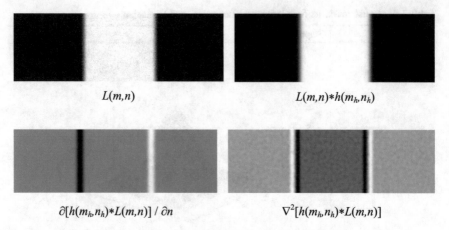

$$L(m,n) \qquad\qquad\qquad L(m,n)*h(m_h,n_h)$$

$$\partial[h(m_h,n_h)*L(m,n)] \,/\, \partial n \qquad\qquad \nabla^2[h(m_h,n_h)*L(m,n)]$$

Fig. 1.4 Input image and image after filtration with the Gauss filter as well as images resulting from the use of different edge detectors after normalization to a range from 0 to 1

$$L_{WG}(m,n) = \nabla^2[h(m_h,n_h) * L(m,n)] \tag{1.14}$$

$$L_{OG}(m,n) = \nabla^2[h(m_h,n_h) * L(m,n)] \tag{1.15}$$

The results obtained with the pre-defined operators (masks) produce satisfactory results in the case of conventional straight edges (Fig. 1.4).

For more complex objects, dedicated algorithms must be applied which detect the edge (edges) and allow for its proper medical interpretation. The extension of this approach and dedicated algorithms will be presented in subsequent chapters of this monograph.

1.4.4 Methods for Assessing the Quality of Edge Detectors

The edge is properly detected when the position of all its points, pixels, is consistent with the pattern. The pattern is most often determined by:

- a medical specialist—expert,
- medical experts (physicians)—in the case of differences between experts, the mean is taken into account,
- results obtained with another more perfect method, for example, another image analysis and processing method which operates more slowly but is more accurate,
- results obtained with other methods—in the case of differences, the mean is taken into account,
- other methodological grounds resulting from, for example, knowledge concerning the actual object contour—anthropometric data.

The use of the pattern in measurements is extremely important from a practical point of view. This allows for a quantitative assessment of the accuracy of edge detection for each of its pixels. In practice, any deviation which is a difference between the reference edge and the detected one is acceptable at this stage. They are most often measured as an absolute value. Since in this case the deviation can be expressed in units of length, it can be calculated for an image of any resolution. In these cases, the error for the entire detected edge is given as a percentage of the number of pixels for which the difference exceeds the predetermined threshold p_r. The value of the threshold p_r is strongly dependent on the image resolution (the higher the resolution, the larger the threshold) and the anthropometric data and medical evidence (the effect of the measurement error on the diagnostic result). Visualization of the location of sample edges is shown in Fig. 1.5.

Tracing the contour $L_w(n)$ (Fig. 1.5) obtained by a medical specialist in relation to the test contour $L_d(n)$ obtained from the test algorithm, various error values are obtained for different values of the threshold p_r. For example (Fig. 1.5), for the threshold $p_r = 1$ pixel, this threshold is exceeded in 7 columns. It means that using the formula for the measurement error δ_g:

$$\delta_g = \frac{\sum_{n=1}^{N} L_0(n)}{N} \cdot 100\% \tag{1.16}$$

where:

$$L_0(n) = \begin{cases} 1 & \text{if } |L_w(n) - L_d(n)| > p_r \\ 0 & \text{other} \end{cases} \tag{1.17}$$

the error value is 63.6 %.

Fig. 1.5 Schematic diagram of a sample arrangement of individual pixels of the contours and object

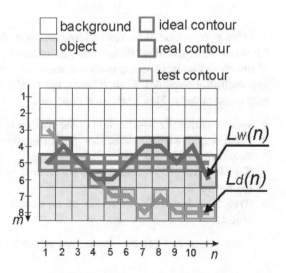

Fig. 1.6 Schematic diagram of a sample arrangement of individual contour pixels in the case of detection of more than one contour for a specific n

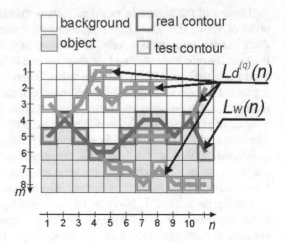

In many practical applications in the medical field, the acceptable error values are significantly tightened up and the threshold p_r is reduced to the resolution error $\pm$ LSB (least significant bit).

In the above discussion it was assumed that the contour $L_d(n)$ obtained from the test algorithm has only one point for each column. In the general case, especially when using Prewitt or Sobel filters, this assumption is not usually met. In this case, a group of q edge portions is obtained, most of which are noise. In such cases, the outermost points of all the contours for a given value n are adopted as the points of the test contour $L_d^{(q)}(n)$. Such situations are shown in Fig. 1.6.

The calculation of the error is modified in this case in the following way:

$$L_0(n) = \begin{cases} 1 & \text{if } \max_q \left| L_w(n) - L_d^{(q)}(n) \right| > p_r \\ 0 & \text{other} \end{cases} \tag{1.18}$$

In the general case, there can be more than one contour, more than one object, on the scene. Such situations occur when, for example, the external or internal contour of the cornea or many corneas on the scene are analysed (if such a situation was hypothetically possible). In such cases, the results of the test algorithm are evaluated quantitatively. This evaluation concerns:

- **False Positive** (*FP*)—detection of the contour in a place where there is no object
- **False Negative** (*FN*)—detection of no object contour in a place where it actually occurs ($\delta_g = 100\ \%$),
- **True Positive** (*TP*)—detection of the contour in a place where it actually occurs ($\delta_g \leq 100\ \%$),
- **True Negative** (*FN*)—detection of no contour in a place where there is no object.

These parameters can be summarized as shown in Table 1.5.

Table 1.5 Definitions of quality parameters of matching the edge

		Edges or objects in the reference image	
		Present (+)	Absent (−)
Edges or objects in the image in the test algorithm	Present (+)	TP	FP
	Absent (−)	FN	TN

Fig. 1.7 Examples of objects with marked ideal contours and contours from the test algorithm as well as indicators *TP*, *FP* and *FN*

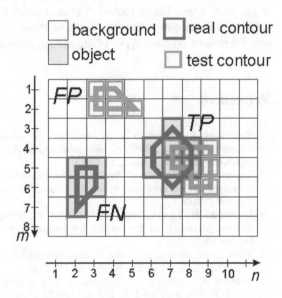

Figure 1.7 shows sample results for the discussed parameters *TP*, *FP* and *FN*. On this basis (Table 1.5), the following parameters have been defined:

- the percentage of matching, touching the edges or objects (sensitivity-**true positive rate**) *TPR*:

$$TPR = \frac{TP}{TP + FN} \cdot 100\% \qquad (1.19)$$

- the coefficient being the measure of the ability to verify the absence of an object or edge (specificity-**true negative rate**) *SPC*:

$$SPC = \frac{TN}{TN + FP} \cdot 100\% \qquad (1.20)$$

- accuracy (**accuracy**-*ACC*)

$$ACC = \frac{TP + TN}{TP + TN + FP + FN} \cdot 100\% \tag{1.21}$$

Changes in sensitivity and specificity when changing algorithm parameters are usually shown on the ROC curves (Receiver Operating Characteristic Curves) and as the AUC (Area Under Curve). The area under the curve is a quantitative indicator of the detector efficiency. Both of these methods enable to compare the effectiveness of different types of algorithms including classifiers.

References

1. Koprowski, R., Ambrósio Jr., R., Reisdorf, S.: Scheimpflug camera in the quantitative assessment of reproducibility of high-speed corneal deformation during intraocular pressure measurement. J. Biophoton. **1**, 11 (2015)
2. Koprowski, R., Kasprzak, H., Wróbel, Z.: New automatic method for analysis and correction of image data from the Corvis tonometer. Comput. Methods Biomech. Biomed. Eng. Imaging Vis. 1–9 (2014)
3. Koprowski, R., Lyssek-Boron, A., Nowinska, A., Wylegala, E., Kasprzak, H., Wróbel, Z.: Selected parameters of the corneal deformation in the Corvis tonometer. BioMed. Eng. OnLine **13**, 55 (2014)
4. Elsheikh, A., Alhasso, D., Rama, P.: Assessment of the epithelium's contribution to corneal biomechanics. Exp. Eye Res. **86**(2), 445–451 (2008)
5. Elsheikh, A., Anderson, K.: Comparative study of corneal strip extensometry and inflation tests. J. R. Soc. Interface **2**(3), 177–185 (2005)
6. Ambrósio, R., Ramos, I., Luz, A., Faria, F., Steinmueller, A., Krug, M., Belin, M., Roberts, C. J.: Dynamic ultra high speed Scheimpflug imaging for assessing corneal biomechanical properties. Revista Brasileira de Oftalmologia **72**(2), 99–102 (2013)
7. Correia, F.F., Ramos, I., Roberts, C.J., Steinmueller, A., Krug, M., Ambrósio Jr., R.: Impact of chamber pressure on the deformation response of corneal models measured by dynamic ultra-high-speed Scheimpflug imaging. Arq. Bras. Oftalmol. **76**(5), 278–281 (2013)
8. Han, Z., Tao, C., Zhou, D., Sun, Y., Zhou, C., Ren, Q., Roberts, C.J.: Air puff induced corneal vibrations: theoretical simulations and clinical observations. J. Refract. Surg. **30**(3), 208–213 (2014)
9. Huseynova, T., Waring 4th, G.O., Roberts, C., Krueger, R.R., Tomita, M.: Corneal biomechanics as a function of intraocular pressure and pachymetry by dynamic infrared signal and Scheimpflug imaging analysis in normal eyes. Am. J. Ophthalmol. **157**(4), 885–893 (2014)
10. Kotecha, A., Elsheikh, A., Roberts, C.R., Zhu, H.G., Garway-Heath, D.F.: Corneal thickness and age-related biomechanical properties of the cornea measured with the ocular response analyzer. Invest. Ophthalmol. Vis. Sci. **47**(12), 5337–5347 (2006)
11. Metzler, K.M., Mahmoud, A.M., Liu, J., Roberts, C.J.: Deformation response of paired donor corneas to an air puff: intact whole globe versus mounted corneoscleral rim. J. Cataract Refract. Surg. **40**(6), 888–896 (2014)
12. Pepose, J.S., Feigenbaum, S.K., Qazi, M.A., Sanderson, J.P., Roberts, C.J.: Changes in corneal biomechanics and intraocular pressure following LASIK using static, dynamic, and noncontact tonometry. Am. J. Ophthalmol. **143**(1), 39–47 (2007)

13. Touboul, D., Roberts, C., Kerautret, J., Garra, C., Maurice-Tison, S., Saubusse, E., Colin, J.: Correlation between corneal hysteresis intraocular pressure, and corneal central pachymetry. J. Cataract Refract. Surg. **34**(4), 616–622 (2008)

14. Valbon, B.F., Ambrósio Jr., R., Fontes, B.M., Luz, A., Roberts, C.J., Alves, M.R.: Ocular biomechanical metrics by CorVis ST in healthy Brazilian patients. J. Refract. Surg. **30**(7), 468–473 (2014)

15. Kling, S.: Corneal biomechanics: measurement, modification and simulation. Ph.D. thesis, University of Valladolid, Spain (2014)

16. Brown, K.E., Congdon, N.G.: Corneal structure and biomechanics: impact on the diagnosis and management of glaucoma. Curr. Opin. Ophthalmol. **17**(4), 338–343 (2006)

17. Dupps, W.J., Wilson, S.E.: Biomechanics and wound healing in the cornea. Exp. Eye Res. **83** (4), 709–720 (2006)

18. Fontes, B.M., Ambrosio Jr., R., Alonso, R.S., Jardim, D., Velarde, G.C., Nose, W.: Corneal biomechanical metrics in eyes with refraction of −19.00 to +9.00 D in healthy Brazilian patients. J. Refract. Surg. **24**(9), 941–945 (2008)

19. Hassan, Z., Modis Jr., L., Szalai, E., Berta, A., Nemeth, G.: Examination of ocular biomechanics with a new Scheimpflug technology after corneal refractive surgery. Cont. Lens Anterior Eye. **37**(5), 337–341 (2014)

20. Kotecha, A.: What biomechanical properties of the cornea are relevant for the clinician? Surv. Ophthalmol. **52**(2), S109–S114 (2007)

21. Luce, D.A.: Determining in vivo biomechanical properties of the cornea with an ocular response analyzer. J. Cataract Refract. Surg. **31**(1), 156–162 (2005)

22. Maeda, N., Ueki, R., Fuchihata, M., Fujimoto, H., Koh, S., Nishida, K.: Corneal biomechanical properties in 3 corneal transplantation techniques with a dynamic Scheimpflug analyzer. Jpn. J. Ophthalmol. **58**(6), 483–489 (2014)

23. Mastropasqua, L., Calienno, R., Lanzini, M., Colasante, M., Mastropasqua, A., Mattei, P.A., Nubile, M.: Evaluation of corneal biomechanical properties modification after small incision lenticule extraction using Scheimpflug-based noncontact tonometer. Biomed. Res. Int. **2014**, 290619 (2014)

24. Ortiz, D., Pinero, D., Shabayek, M.H., Arnalich-Montiel, F., Alió, J.L.: Corneal biomechanical properties in normal, post-laser in situ keratomileusis, and keratoconic eyes. J. Cataract Refract. Surg. **33**(8), 1371–1375 (2007)

25. Pedersen, I.B., Bak-Nielsen, S., Vestergaard, A.H., Ivarsen, A., Hjortdal, J.: Corneal biomechanical properties after LASIK, ReLEx flex, and ReLEx smile by Scheimpflug-based dynamic tonometry. Graefes Arch. Clin. Exp. Ophthalmol. **252**(8), 1329–1335 (2014)

26. Shah, S., Laiquzzaman, M., Bhojwani, R., Mantry, S., Cunliffe, I.: Assessment of the biomechanical properties of the cornea with the ocular response analyzer in normal and keratoconic eyes. Invest. Ophthalmol. Vis. Sci. **48**(7), 3026–3031 (2007)

27. Shah, S., Laiquzzaman, M., Cunliffe, I., Mantry, S.: The use of the Reichert ocular response analyser to establish the relationship between ocular hysteresis, corneal resistance factor and central corneal thickness in normal eyes. Cont. Lens Anterior Eye **29**(5), 257–262 (2006)

28. Smedowski, A., Weglarz, B., Tarnawska, D., Kaarniranta, K., Wylegala, E.: Comparison of three intraocular pressure measurement methods including biomechanical properties of the cornea. Invest. Ophthalmol. Vis. Sci. **55**(2), 666–673 (2014)

29. Hallahan, K.M., Sinha Roy, A., Ambrosio Jr., R., Salomao, M., Dupps Jr., W.J.: Discriminant value of custom ocular response analyzer waveform derivatives in keratoconus. Ophthalmology **121**(2), 459–468 (2014)

30. Gao, M., Liu, Y., Xiao, Y., Han, G., Jia, L., Wang, L., Lei, T., Huang, Y.: Prolonging survival of corneal transplantation by selective sphingosine-1-phosphate receptor 1 agonist. PLoS ONE **9**(9), e105693 (2014)

31. Lanza, M., Cennamo, M., Iaccarino, S., Irregolare, C., Rechichi, M., Bifani, M., Gironi Carnevale, U.A.: Evaluation of corneal deformation analyzed with Scheimpflug based device in healthy eyes and diseased ones. Biomed. Res. Int. **2014**, 748671 (2014)

32. Shen, Y., Chen, Z., Knorz, M.C., Li, M., Zhao, J., Zhou, X.: Comparison of corneal deformation parameters after SMILE, LASEK, and femtosecond laser-assisted LASIK. J. Refract. Surg. **30**(5), 310–318 (2014)
33. Shen, Y., Zhao, J., Yao, P., Miao, H., Niu, L., Wang, X., Zhou, X.: Changes in corneal deformation parameters after lenticule creation and extraction during small incision lenticule extraction (SMILE) procedure. PLoS ONE **9**(8), e103893 (2014)
34. Marjanović, I., Martinez, A., Marjanović, M., Milić, N., Kontić, D., Hentova-Senćanić, P., Marković, V., Bozić, M.: Changes in the retrobulbar hemodynamic parameters after decreasing the elevated intraocular pressure in primary open-angle glaucoma patients. Srp. Arh. Celok. Lek. **142**(5–6), 286–290 (2014)
35. Papastergiou, G.I., Kozobolis, V., Siganos, D.S.: Effect of recipient corneal pathology on Pascal tonometer and Goldmann tonometer readings in eyes after penetrating keratoplasty. Eur. J. Ophthalmol. **20**(1), 29–34 (2010)
36. Sawada, A., Yamada, H., Yamamoto, Y., Yamamoto, T.: Intraocular pressure alterations after visual field testing. Jpn. J. Ophthalmol. **58**(5), 429–434 (2014)
37. Chunhong, J., Jinhua, Y., Tianjie, L., Lei, T., Yifei, H., Yuanyuan, W., Yongping, Z.: Dynamic curvature topography for evaluating the anterior corneal surface change with Corvis ST. BioMed. Eng. OnLine **14**, 53 (2015)
38. Koprowski, R., Wilczyński, S., Nowinska, A., Lyssek-Boron, A., Teper, S., Wylegala, E., Wróbel, Z.: Quantitative assessment of responses of the eyeball based on data from the Corvis tonometer. Comput. Biol. Med. **58**, 91–100 (2015)
39. Koprowski, R.: Automatic method of analysis and measurement of additional parameters of corneal deformation in the Corvis tonometer. Biomed. Eng. Online **13**, 150 (2014)
40. Gonzalez, R.C., Woods, R.E.: Digital Image Processing, 3rd edn. Prentice Hall: Pearson Education, Inc., Upper Saddle River, New Jersey (2007)

Chapter 2
Image Pre-processing

2.1 Image Acquisition

Image acquisition was carried out in the Corvis tonometer. The results can be exported to various formats directly from the original software (OCULUS Corvis ST ver 1.02r 1126). The following formats have been used in practice:

- *U12*—a compressed file with a database of patients,
- *CST*—a compressed file of one patient,
- **.avi*—an AVI file with a sequence of images of the cornea,
- **.jpg*—a sequence of images in jpg format from *patient's_name_date_000.jpg* to *patient's_name_date_139.jpg*.

A block diagram of the data acquisition and connection, through file conversion, with Matlab is shown in Fig. 2.1.

Later in the monograph the operation of the algorithm individual parts was verified using the Operating System: Microsoft Windows 7 Version 6.1 (Build 7601: Service Pack 1) Java VM Version: Java 1.6.0_17-b04 with Sun Microsystems Inc. Java HotSpot(TM) 64-Bit Server VM mixed mode in Matlab Version 7.11.0.584 (R2010b) with Image Processing Toolbox Version 7.1 (R2010b). The PC computer was equipped with Intel Xeon X5680 @ 3.33 GHz with 12 GB of RAM.

The last two data formats (**.avi* and **.jpg*) are most convenient for data processing. Loading and showing a sequence of images previously saved in the folder *C:/data* in **.jpg* format to Matlab can be done using the following code:

© Springer International Publishing Switzerland 2016

R. Koprowski, *Image Analysis for Ophthalmological Diagnosis*,
Studies in Computational Intelligence 631, DOI 10.1007/978-3-319-29546-6_2

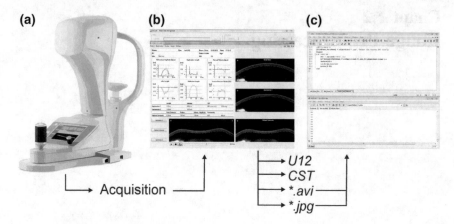

Fig. 2.1 Block diagram of the data acquisition and connection, through file conversion, with Matlab: **a** Corvis tonometer, **b** application OCULUS Corvis ST, **c** Matlab with the algorithm discussed in this monograph

```
cd('C:/data');
[FileName,PathName] = uigetfile('*.jpg','Select the
Corvis JPG file');
figure
for i=0:139
    str = sprintf('%03d',i);
    LG=imread([PathName,FileName(1:end-
7),str,FileName(end-3:end)]);
    imshow(LG);
    title(mat2str(i))
    pause(0.01)
end
```

Function *cd* is designed to set the path, *uigetfile* function enables to open a dialog where the user can select any **.jpg* file from the image sequence. The file selection is followed by sequential reading of successive *jpg* images from $i = 0$ to $i = 139$. With the use of *sprintf* function it is possible to convert the value i to an appropriate string form, "000" instead of "0", "001" instead of "1" etc. *Imread* function enables to load the appropriate file to the matrix L_G. Next, functions title and *mat2str* enable to show the image number in its header. With *pause* function it is possible to delay the loop operation due to the need to display individual images from a sequence.

In the case of *.avi* file, the following notation can be used:

```
cd('C:/data');
[FileName,PathName] = uigetfile('*.avi','Select the Cor-
vis AVI file');
Obj = mmreader([PathName,FileName]);
figure
for i=1:Obj.NumberOfFrames
    LGi = read(Obj, i);
    imshow(LGi);
    title(mat2str(i))
    pause(0.01)
end
```

Function *mmreader* (*aviread* in older versions of Matlab) enables to download the movie file handle. Then *read* function allows for loading individual frames as 2D images.

In this loop, and also in the previous one, it is possible to perform three basic tasks useful for further analysis:

- visualization of an image sequence—as it has been done in the presented source code,
- saving an image sequence as subsequent files with the extension *.mat*,
- saving an image sequence as one file in the Matlab data format—*.mat*.

The choice of the appropriate method depends on the direction of further analysis. As the essential elements in further analysis are the cornea and its contour, saving all the images on the disk in the form of one matrix is not necessary. Additionally, the creation of one matrix containing the full sequence of 140 images occupies in the Matlab space 16,128,000 bytes for data in *uint8* format ($M \times N \times I = 200 \times 576 \times 140$ pixels). Compared to a single 2D image, it is 115,200 bytes in *uint8* format ($M \times N = 200 \times 576$ pixels).

The subsequent images loaded into Matlab will be the variable L_G. The notation $L_G(m, n)$, where m—row coordinates, n—column coordinates, will be used equally often. Later in the monograph, other variables will be indexed at the bottom in accordance with the notation of the following image matrices for subsequent analysis phases. In the notation of source codes in Matlab, subscripts and superscripts will be replaced with normal letters. In addition, readers who will not use the *m*-files added to the monograph should pay attention to too long strings which were divided between the text lines. This division is important because the division between the lines in the source code in Matlab is marked with an ellipsis "…". However, it is not included in this monograph.

2.2   Image Filtration

Immediately after loading the image L_G into Matlab, noise and small artefacts were filtered. Initial analyses confirmed that the greatest distortions, when taking proper care of the tonometer optics (its purity), are clusters consisting of no more than 3, 4 pixels. In this case, the median filter is the best option due to its characteristics, mainly the ability to remove impulse noise. The available function representing the median filter is *medfilt2*. In addition, the size of the mask h_1 is given, namely $M_{h1} \times N_{h1}$. This is the size of the window within which the median will be calculated. Since, as mentioned earlier, distortions are clusters that do not exceed 4 pixels, the sufficient size of the median filter mask is $M_{h1} \times N_{h1} = 3 \times 3$ pixels— because $4 < (M_{h1} \cdot N_{h1})/2$. In practice, this provides 9 pixels, from which the middle one is chosen after sorting. With *imnoise* function, it is possible to trace the relationship between the level of distortions (image L_{NO}) and the results obtained from median filtering—image L_{MED}. For a sample image for $i = 70$ and the selected area, $m \in (80, 120)$, $n \in (80, 120)$:

```
cd('C:/data');
[FileName,PathName] = uigetfile('*.jpg','Select the Cor-
vis JPG file');
i=70;
str = sprintf('%03d',i);
LG=imread([PathName,FileName(1:end-7),str,FileName(end-
3:end)]);
for d=0.01:0.2:0.61
    LNO=imnoise(LG,'salt & pepper',d);
    figure; imshow(LNO);
     axis([80 120 80 120])

    xlabel('n
[pixel]','FontSize',20,'FontAngle','Italic');
    ylabel('m
[pixel]','FontSize',20,'FontAngle','Italic');
    LMED=medfilt2(LNO,[3 3],'symmetric');
    figure; imshow(LMED);
     axis([80 120 80 120])
    xlabel('n
[pixel]','FontSize',20,'FontAngle','Italic');
    ylabel('m
[pixel]','FontSize',20,'FontAngle','Italic');
end
```

The value d is noise density and $d \in \{0.01, 0.21, 0.41, 0.61\}$. The results obtained can be traced in Fig. 2.2.

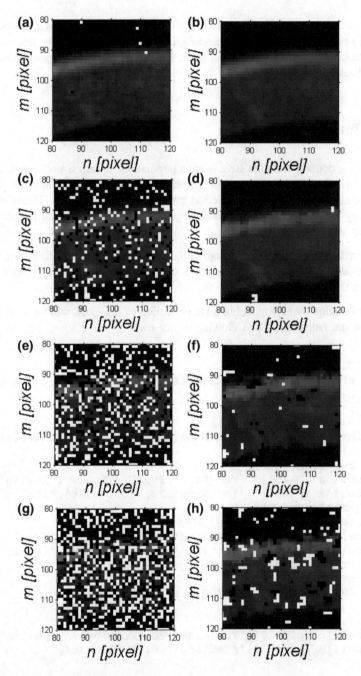

Fig. 2.2 Image sequence obtained for different *d* values (noise density) of noise added to the image L_G. The following images show the portion of the image L_{NO} with noise (*first column*) and the image L_{MED} after median filtering (*second column*) for: **a**, **b** *d* = 0.01, **c**, **d** *d* = 0.21, **e**, **f** *d* = 0.41, **g**, **h** *d* = 61

The image sequence (presented in Fig. 2.2) obtained for different *d* values (noise density) of noise added to the image L_G confirms, in all cases, the necessity and reasonableness of using the median filter. The next step of image pre-processing is normalization.

2.3 Image Normalization

Images L_G coming from different human populations obtained under various conditions are characterized by various parameters relating to brightness. In general, these images have a histogram shifted towards the darker pixels. Therefore, it is necessary to carry out normalization. Image normalization can be carried out in two different ways:

- normalization of the entire image to the range of brightness values from 0 to 1,
- normalization of individual columns or rows to a range of brightness values from 0 to 1.

The function *mat2gray*, being a simplification of *imadjust*, will be used in both types of normalization. The following source code:

```
cd('C:/data');
[FileName,PathName] = uigetfile('*.jpg','Select the Cor-
vis JPG file');
i=70;
str = sprintf('%03d',i);
LG=imread([PathName,FileName(1:end-7),str,FileName(end-
3:end)]);
figure; imshow(LG);
xlabel('n [pixel]','FontSize',20,'FontAngle','Italic');
ylabel('m [pixel]','FontSize',20,'FontAngle','Italic');
LRM1=mat2gray(LG);
figure; imshow(LRM1);
xlabel('n [pixel]','FontSize',20,'FontAngle','Italic');
ylabel('m [pixel]','FontSize',20,'FontAngle','Italic');
LRM2=zeros(size(LG));
for n=1:size(LG,2)
    LRM2(:,n)=mat2gray(LG(:,n));
end
figure; imshow(LRM2);
xlabel('n [pixel]','FontSize',20,'FontAngle','Italic');
ylabel('m [pixel]','FontSize',20,'FontAngle','Italic');
```

provides the results shown in the image in Fig. 2.3.

In general and also in the analysed case (Fig. 2.3), normalization with the first method is more often used. This is due to the fact that the relationships between

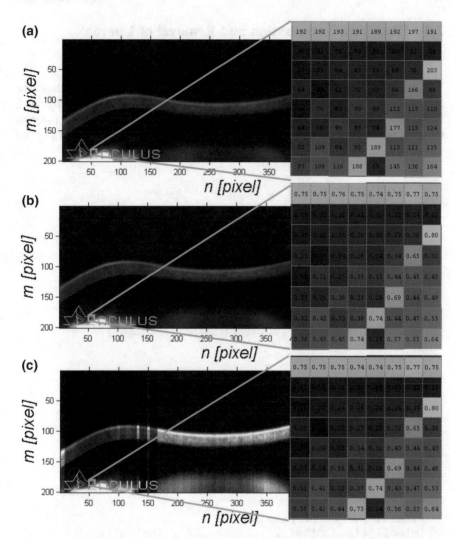

Fig. 2.3 Image L_G (**a**) and images L_{RM} after normalization with the first method (**b**) and the second method (**c**) as well as the zoom of their selected fragment

pixels remain unchanged. Subsequent columns are modified in a linear manner. The results obtained with the second normalization method are much more impressive. However, their usefulness in practice, as will be shown in the following chapters, is smaller.

2.4 Histogram Equalization and Removal of Uneven Background

The next step is histogram equalization, partly related to the normalization discussed in the previous subchapter, and the removal of uneven background. Histogram equalization is reduced to the use of *histeq* function and the function intended to visualize the histogram, namely *imhist*. The results provided in Fig. 2.4 were obtained using the source code shown below.

```
figure; imshow(LG);
xlabel('n
[pixel]','FontSize',20,'FontAngle','Italic');
ylabel('m
[pixel]','FontSize',20,'FontAngle','Italic');
figure; imhist(LG)
text('Units','normalized','Position',[0.4,-
0.16],'String','intensity','FontSize',20,'FontAngle','
Italic');
ylabel('number of pixels
[pixel]','FontSize',20,'FontAngle','Italic');
grid on

LQ=histeq(LG);
figure; imshow(LQ);
xlabel('n
[pixel]','FontSize',20,'FontAngle','Italic');
ylabel('m
[pixel]','FontSize',20,'FontAngle','Italic');
figure; imhist(LQ)
text('Units','normalized','Position',[0.4,-
0.16],'String','intensity','FontSize',20,'FontAngle','
Italic');
ylabel('number of pixels
[pixel]','FontSize',20,'FontAngle','Italic');
grid on
```

Figure 2.4 shows the image L_G and its histogram as well as the image after histogram equalization L_Q together with its histogram.

Histogram equalization shown in Fig. 2.4 significantly increases the contrast between adjacent pixels. The corneal contour is more visible. Non-uniformity of brightness for the rows from 1 to about 90 is also visible. It is illustrated in the graph in Fig. 2.5.

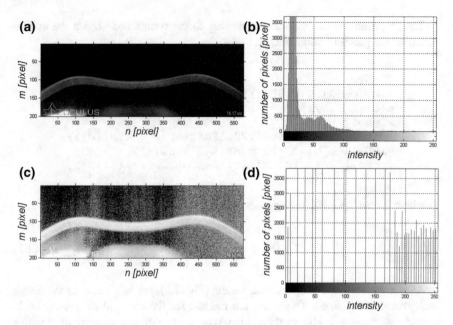

Fig. 2.4 Image L_G (**a**), and its histogram (**b**), image after histogram equalization L_Q (**d**), and its histogram

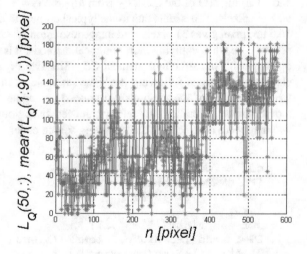

Fig. 2.5 Graph of brightness changes for a sample row $m = 50$ (*red*) and the average range for $m \in (1.90)$ (*green*), the image after histogram equalization L_Q

The graph above was obtained according to the source code being the contin-uation of the previous fragment, i.e.:

```
figure;
plot(mean(LQ(1:90,:)),'-g*'); hold on; grid on
plot(LQ(50,:),'-r*');
xlabel('n
[pixel]','FontSize',20,'FontAngle','Italic');
ylabel('L_Q(50,:), mean(L_Q(1:90,:))
[pixel]','FontSize',20,'FontAngle','Italic');
```

where *mean(LQ(1:90,:))* expresses the value of the variable L_{QS}, i.e.:

$$L_{QS}(n) = \frac{1}{91} \cdot \sum_{m=1}^{m=90} L_Q(m,n) \qquad (2.1)$$

As is apparent from the presented results (Fig. 2.5), the brightness of the image background is not fixed. Therefore, the method for the removal of uneven back-ground was proposed. This method is based on the use of an averaging filter with a large mask size or morphological methods also with a large size of the structural element.

In the first case this is the convolution operation expressed by the relation (1.8) and a varying size of the mask h_2, from $M_{h2} \times N_{h2} = 31 \times 31$ pixels to $M_{h2} \times N_{h2} = 90 \times 90$ pixels. This size is due to the typical corneal thickness of 500 μm, which at 16.5 μm/pixel gives 31 pixels, and image resolution $M \times N = 200 \times 576$ pixels. In the second case when applying morphological methods, it is most often the operation of opening with the structural element SE_1. The size $M_{SE1} \times N_{SE1}$ of the structural element was chosen following the same rationale as in the selection of the mask size in the case of the previously discussed averaging filter. The results of using morphological operations to remove uneven background are shown in Fig. 2.6 and they were obtained for the following source code:

```
cd('C:/data');
[FileName,PathName] = uigetfile('*.jpg','Select the
Corvis JPG file');
i=70;
str = sprintf('%03d',i);
LG=imread([PathName,FileName(1:end-
7),str,FileName(end-3:end)]);
LCS=[];
```

```
for MSE1=[1 11 21 31 91]
    NSE1=MSE1;
    SE1=ones([MSE1 NSE1]);
    LO=imopen(LG,SE1);
    LC=abs(LG-LO);
    figure; imshow(histeq(LC))
    xlabel('n
[pixel]','FontSize',20,'FontAngle','Italic');
    ylabel('m
[pixel]','FontSize',20,'FontAngle','Italic');
    LCS=[LCS,mean(LC(1:90,:))'];
end
figure;
plot(LCS);   grid on
xlabel('n
[pixel]','FontSize',20,'FontAngle','Italic');
ylabel('L_{CS}(n)
[pixel]','FontSize',20,'FontAngle','Italic');
legend('1x1','11x11','21x21','31x31','91x91')
```

The results shown in Figs. 2.6 and 2.7 refer to the image L_G with adjusted uneven lighting, i.e.:

$$L_C(m,n) = |L_G(m,n) - L_O(m,n)| \qquad (2.2)$$

where:

$$L_O(m,n) = \max_{SE1}\left(\min_{SE1} L_G(m,n)\right) \qquad (2.3)$$

and the value L_{CS} defined as:

$$L_{CS}(n) = \frac{1}{91} \cdot \sum_{m=1}^{m=90} L_C(m,n) \qquad (2.4)$$

The graph presented in Fig. 2.7 shows that the smallest background brightness changes are for the structural element sized $M_{SE1} \times N_{SE1} = 11 \times 11$ pixels. However, this value of the structural element size causes degradation of the cornea (Fig. 2.6a). The optimum values are therefore the structural element sizes in the range $M_{SE1} = N_{SE1} \in (11, 21)$ pixels. Evidence of this is the analysis of the brightness of the image section—for the selected column of the image L_C, for example, for 100 pixels—Fig. 2.8.

The graphs in Fig. 2.8 reach the highest dynamics for $M_{SE1} \times N_{SE1} = 31 \times 31$ and $M_{SE1} \times N_{SE1} = 91 \times 91$ pixels. However, only for the former mask size ($M_{SE1} \times N_{SE1} = 31 \times 31$ pixels) the background brightness for $m \in (120, 160)$ pixels is comparable with the results obtained for the smaller size of the structural

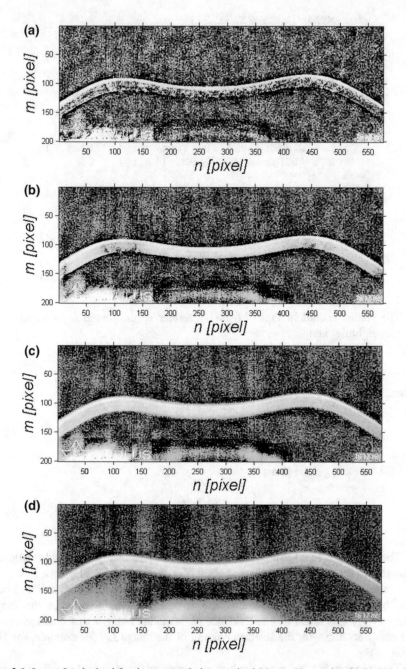

Fig. 2.6 Image L_C obtained for the structural element sized $M_{SEI} \times N_{SEI} \in \{11\ 21\ 31\ 91\}$ after histogram equalization: **a** for 11×11 pixels, **b** for 21×21 pixels, **c** for 31×31 pixels and **d** for 91×91 pixels

Fig. 2.7 Graphs L_{CS} for the image L_C with uneven background correction at $M_{SE1} \times N_{SE1} = 1 \times 1$ pixel (no correction), 11×11, 21×21, 31×31 and 91×91 pixels

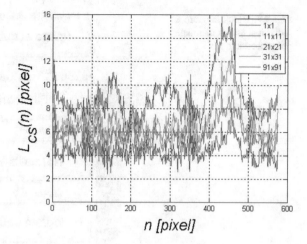

Fig. 2.8 Graphs of brightness changes for the column number 100 of the image L_C at $M_{SE1} \times N_{SE1} = 1 \times 1$ pixel (no correction), 11×11, 21×21, 31×31 and 91×91 pixels

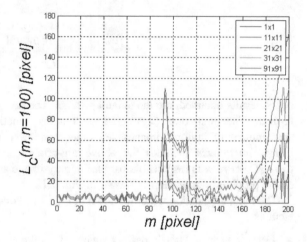

elements (it does not exceed 10 Fig. 2.8). Therefore, when removing uneven background from the images L_G, morphological opening operations with a structural element sized $M_{SE1} \times N_{SE1} = 31 \times 31$ pixels were used.

2.5   Summary of Image Pre-processing

The individual blocks of image pre-processing discussed in the previous sub-chapters are shown in Fig. 2.9

The whole discussed image pre-processing algorithm has been provided in the form of a graphical user interface (GUI). The individual values of masks and structural elements are those parameters that are set by the user. The best, in terms

Fig. 2.9 Block diagram of
individual stages of image
pre-processing

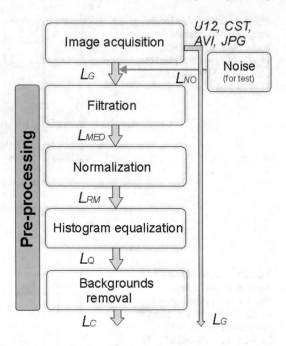

of the results obtained, are the default settings. The designed GUI consists of three
m-files. The first one *CorvisGUI.m* contains functions responsible for the
arrangement of buttons, images and other windows. The second m-file named
CorvisFunctions.m includes the above pre-processing stages. The third m-file
CorvisCalcPre.m is responsible for preliminary image analysis. The main window
of the proposed application is shown in Fig. 2.10.

The main application window shown in Fig. 2.10 consists of a few characteristic
elements:

- *Default menu*—Matlab default menu, it includes image recording, reading,
  printing, changing the settings of menu items and so on.
- *Main menu*—menu created for pre-processing of images from the Corvis
  tonometer. It includes:

  - *Open*—button intended to point to *avi* or *jpg* files containing a sequence of
    images
  - *ReCal*—button responsible for the recalculation of parameters for a full
    sequence of *i* images.
  - *MedFilter*—textbox—non-editable—median filtering.
  - *3 × 3*—sample setting from the drop-down menu associated with the size of
    the mask h_1 during median filtering. The following settings are possible:
    "*None|3 × 3|7 × 7|9 × 9|11 × 11|15 × 15|23 × 23*"
  - *Normal*—textbox—non-editable—normalization.

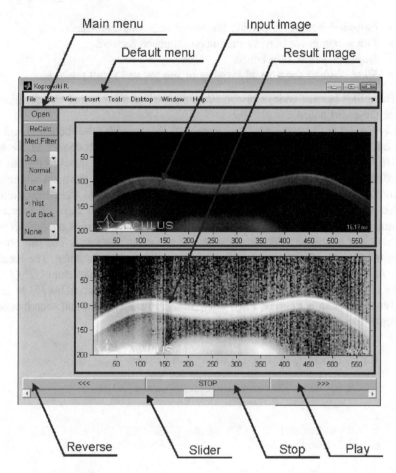

Fig. 2.10 Main application window (GUI)

- *Local*—one of the settings of the drop-down menu associated with normalization. The following settings are possible: "*None|Global|Local*"
- *Hist*—radio button designed to indicate whether histogram equalization was or was not performed in the image.
- *Cut. Back.*—textbox—non-editable—cut background.
- *None*—one of the settings of the drop-down menu associated with background removal. The following settings are possible: "*None|21 × 21| 27 × 27|31 × 31|37 × 37|45 × 45*"

- *Input image*—input image L_G.
- *Result image*—result image as the result of analysis, in this case, the result of image pre-processing. In the general case, it is the result of image pre-processing and main processing (see Fig. 2.9).

- *Reverse*—button for playing the image sequence backwards.
- *Play*—button for playing the image sequence forward.
- *Stop*—playback stop button
- *Slider*—slider for manual viewing of images and result analysis.

Three files (source code) *CorvisGUI.m, CorvisFunctions.m* and *CorvisCalcPre. m* are presented below.

CorvisGUI.m file consists of a commentary that provides the file name and the last update. These data are displayed after calling the Matlab command >> *help corvisGUI* in the main window. The second part of the file mostly contains the function *uicontrol* designed for embedding the menu items in the main window—*figure*. The first code line (after the comment "%") relates to the declaration of global variables. This is the variable *hObj* carrying, in the form of a matrix, information about handles to individual menu items. Then there is the default path to the folder containing the sample data—in this case *"C:/data"*. The subsequent paths are the use of *uicontrol* function to create the next menu items. The handles from *hObj(2)* to *hObj(10)* concern *main menu* (Fig. 2.10), handles from *hObj(11)* to *hObj(15)* concern *Input image* and *Result image*, handles from *hObj(15)* to *hObj (18)* concern buttons *Reverse, Play, Stop, Slider* (Fig. 2.10). The full source code is presented below.

```
%CorvisGUI graphical user interface
%
%    See also CorvisFunction CorvisCalcPre
%    Copyright 2015 Robert Koprowski
%
%    $Revision: 2.1 $  $Date: 2015/07/09 10:40:11 $
global hObj

cd('C:/data');
path='C:/data';

hObj(1)=figure('Name','Koprowski
R.','NumberTitle','off');
col=get(hObj(1),'Color')*0.9;
```

```
hObj(2)=uicontrol('Style', 'pushbut-
ton','units','normalized','FontUnits','normalized',
'String', 'Open',    'Position', [0.001 0.95 0.1
0.05],'Callback', 'CorvisFunc-
tion(1)','BackgroundColor',col);
hObj(3)=uicontrol('Style', 'pushbut-
ton','units','normalized','FontUnits','normalized',
'String', 'ReCalc',    'Position', [0.001 0.9 0.1
0.05],'Callback', 'CorvisFunc-
tion(2)','BackgroundColor',col);
hObj(4)=uicontrol('Style',
'text','units','normalized','FontUnits','normalized','
String', 'Med.Filter','Value',3,'Position', [0.001
0.85 0.1 0.05],'BackgroundColor',col);
hObj(5)=uicontrol('Style',
'popup','units','normalized','FontUnits','normalized',
'String',
'None|3x3|7x7|9x9|11x11|15x15|23x23','Value',3,'Positi
on', [0.001 0.8 0.1
0.05],'Callback','CorvisFunction(3)','BackgroundColor'
,col);
hObj(6)=uicontrol('Style',
'text','units','normalized','FontUnits','normalized','
String', 'Normal.','Value',3,'Position', [0.001 0.75
0.1 0.05],'BackgroundColor',col);
hObj(7)=uicontrol('Style',
'popup','units','normalized','FontUnits','normalized',
'String', 'None|Global|Local','Value',3,'Position',
[0.001 0.7 0.1
0.05],'Callback','CorvisFunction(4)','BackgroundColor'
,col);
```

```
hObj(8)=uicontrol('Style', 'radiobut-
ton','units','normalized','FontUnits','normalized','St
ring', 'hist','Value',1,'Position', [0.001 0.65 0.1
0.05],'Callback','CorvisFunction(5)','BackgroundColor'
,col);
hObj(9)=uicontrol('Style',
'text','units','normalized','FontUnits','normalized','
String', 'Cut Back.','Value',2,'Position', [0.001 0.6
0.1 0.05],'BackgroundColor',col);
hObj(10)=uicontrol('Style',
'popup','units','normalized','FontUnits','normalized',
'String',
'None|21x21|27x27|31x31|37x37|45x45','Value',4,'Positi
on', [0.001 0.55 0.1
0.05],'Callback','CorvisFunction(6)','BackgroundColor'
,col);

hObj(11)=axes('Parent',hObj(1),'units','normalized','P
osition', [0.2 0.52 0.78 0.45]);
hObj(12)=imshow(rand(200,576),'InitialMagnification','
fit','Parent',hObj(11)); hold on
hObj(13)=axes('Parent',hObj(1),'units','normalized','P
osition', [0.2 0.1 0.78 0.45]);
hObj(14)=imshow(rand(200,576),'InitialMagnification','
fit','Parent',hObj(13)); hold on

hObj(15)=uicontrol('Style',
'slider','units','normalized','FontUnits','normalized'
,'BackgroundColor',col,'Position', [0.001 0.01 0.999
0.03],'Min',0,'Max',139,'Value',0,'Callback', 'Corvis-
Function(7)');
hObj(16)=uicontrol('Style', 'pushbut-
ton','units','normalized','FontUnits','normalized',
'String', '<<<',  'Position', [0.001 0.04 0.35
0.04],'Callback', 'CorvisFunc-
tion(8)','BackgroundColor',col);
hObj(17)=uicontrol('Style', 'pushbut-
ton','units','normalized','FontUnits','normalized',
'String', 'STOP','Position', [0.351 0.04 0.349
0.04],'Callback', 'CorvisFunc-
tion(9)','BackgroundColor',col);
hObj(18)=uicontrol('Style', 'pushbut-
ton','units','normalized','FontUnits','normalized',
'String', '>>>','Position', [0.70 0.04 0.3
0.04],'Callback', 'CorvisFunc-
tion(10)','BackgroundColor',col);
```

The second file *CorvisFunction.m* relates to action that is taken when pressing any button or selecting any item from *Main menu*. The function argument is a variable *sw* which is dependent on the element from *Main menu* which was selected with a mouse or pressed—it is linked with, e.g. notation, as in the case of the slider *'Callback', 'CorvisFunction(7)'* (see the source code above). Any *avi* or *jpg* file is read by opening the window intended for the file selection using *uigetfile* function and then reading the image sequence. In the case of the sequence of *jpg* images, it was assumed, according to the data obtained directly from the Corvis tonometer, that they are numbered from **000.jpg* to **139.jpg*. In another case or in the absence of any file, Matlab will report an error. For images saved as subsequent frames of *avi* video, all the available frames are read, regardless of their number—see the variable *aviObj.NumberOfFrames*. At this point I encourage readers to test the program thoroughly and to create their own security. For example, information can be shown to the operator in the absence of the full sequence of *jpg* files or in the case of incorrect image resolution, e.g. using the function *warndlg*. The source code of the discussed CorvisFunction is shown below:

```
function []=CorvisFunction(sw)
global hObj PathName FileName break_ LGi LMED LRM LQ
LC h1 Norm Hist MSE1
if (sw==1)|(sw==2) % OPEN OR RECALCULATION
    if sw==1 % if OPEN
        [FileName,PathName] = uiget-
file('*.jpg;*.avi','Select the Corvis JPG or AVI
file');
    end
    if FileName~=0 % if select file
        if strcmp(FileName(end-
2:end),'jpg')|strcmp(FileName(end-2:end),'JPG')
            set(hObj(14),'CData',rand(200,576))
            for i=0:139
                str = sprintf('%03d',i);

                LGi=imread([PathName,FileName(1:end-
7),str,FileName(end-3:end)]);
                LGi=double(LGi)/255;
                set(hObj(12),'CData',LGi);
                set(hObj(15),'Value',i);
                set(hObj(15),'Max',139,'Min',0);
                CorvisFunction(3);
                pause(0.01)

            end
```

```
        elseif strcmp(FileName(end-2:end),'avi')
            set(hObj(14),'CData',rand(200,576))
            aviObj = mmreader([PathName,FileName]);
            for i=1:aviObj.NumberOfFrames
                LGi = read(aviObj, i);
                LGi=double(LGi(:,:,1))/255;
                set(hObj(12),'CData',LGi);
                set(hObj(15),'Value',i);

    set(hObj(15),'Max',aviObj.NumberOfFrames,'Min',1);
                CorvisFunction(3);
                pause(0.01)
            end
        else
            FileName(end-2:end)
            disp('Please select AVI or JPG')
        end
    end
end
```

Subsequent parts of *CorvisFunction* relate to assigning values to variables *h1, Norm, Hist, MSE*. The values are selected by the user by means of the drop-down menu. This drop-down menu has values of the variable *sw* equal to 3, 4, 5 or 6. Accordingly:

- *h1* is the mask size of the averaging filter,
- *Norm* is the variable indicating whether normalization needs to be performed, or whether normalization should be local or global,
- *Hist* is the variable indicating whether histogram equalization needs to be performed or not,
- *MSE1* is the size of the structural element necessary to remove uneven background, this element is always square with a declared number of rows and columns.

The source code responsible for this part is given below:

```
if (sw==3)|(sw==4)|(sw==5)|(sw==6)
% MEDIAN None|3x3|7x7|9x9|11x11|15x15|23x23
    if get(hObj(5),'Value')==1
        h1=0;
    end
    if get(hObj(5),'Value')==2
        h1=3;
    end
    if get(hObj(5),'Value')==3
        h1=7;
    end
    if get(hObj(5),'Value')==4
        h1=9;
    end
    if get(hObj(5),'Value')==5
        h1=11;
    end
    if get(hObj(5),'Value')==6
        h1=15;
    end
    if get(hObj(5),'Value')==7
        h1=23;
    end
% normalization %None|Global|Local
    if get(hObj(7),'Value')==1
        Norm=0;
    end
    if get(hObj(7),'Value')==2
        Norm=1;
    end
    if get(hObj(7),'Value')==3
        Norm=2;
    end
% Hist %None|HIST
    Hist=get(hObj(8),'Value');
%Backgroung %None|21x21|27x27|31x31|37x37|45x45
    if get(hObj(10),'Value')==1
        MSE1=0;
    end
    if get(hObj(10),'Value')==2
        MSE1=21;
    end
    if get(hObj(10),'Value')==3
        MSE1=27;
    end
    if get(hObj(10),'Value')==4
        MSE1=31;
    end
```

```
      if get(hObj(10),'Value')==5
          MSE1=37;
      end
      if get(hObj(10),'Value')==6
          MSE1=45;
      end
%%%%%%%%%%%%%%%%%%%%%%%%%%%%%%%%%%%%%%%%%%%%%%%%%%%%%%%%

[LMED,LRM,LQ,LC]=CorvisCalcPre(LGi,h1,Norm,Hist,MSE1);
          set(hObj(14),'CData',LC);


end
```

The last part of the code contains a reference to the function *CorvisCalcPre* which is responsible for performing computations in the image *LGi* (*i*-th input image). The last part of the discussed source code of the function *CorvisFunction* relates to navigation while browsing back and forth the images before and after image pre-processing. At the end of each loop and performed calculations (*CorvisCalcPre* function), there is *pause* function with a parameter (0.01 s) which refers to the time needed to display an image. In the absence of the *pause* function, the last image in the performed loop will be displayed (*for*). This function fragment includes another variable *break_* which is the flag directly related to pressing the *Stop* button. The *set* functions refresh the image and other parameters according to their calculated values.

```
      if sw==7 % SLIDER
          i=round(get(hObj(15),'Value'));
          if strcmp(FileName(end-
2:end),'jpg')|strcmp(FileName(end-2:end),'JPG')
              str = sprintf('%03d',i);
              LGi=imread([PathName,FileName(1:end-
7),str,FileName(end-3:end)]);
              LGi=double(LGi)/255;
              set(hObj(12),'CData',LGi);
          elseif strcmp(FileName(end-2:end),'avi')
              aviObj = mmreader([PathName,FileName]);
              LGi = read(aviObj, i);
              LGi=double(LGi(:,:,1))/255;
              set(hObj(12),'CData',LGi);
          else
              disp('Please select AVI or JPG')
          end
          CorvisFunction(3);
      end
      if sw==8 % <<<<<<<<<<<<<
```

```
          if strcmp(FileName(end-
2:end),'jpg')|strcmp(FileName(end-2:end),'JPG')
              for i=round(get(hObj(15),'Value')):-1:0
                  str = sprintf('%03d',i);
                  LGi=imread([PathName,FileName(1:end-
7),str,FileName(end-3:end)]);
                  LGi=double(LGi)/255;
                  set(hObj(12),'CData',LGi);
                  set(hObj(15),'Value',i);
                  set(hObj(15),'Max',139,'Min',0);
                  CorvisFunction(3);
                  if break_==1
                      break_=0;
                      break
                  end
                  pause(0.01)

              end
          elseif strcmp(FileName(end-2:end),'avi')
              aviObj = mmreader([PathName,FileName]);
              for i=round(get(hObj(15),'Value')):-1:1
                  LGi = read(aviObj, i);
                  LGi=double(LGi(:,:,1))/255;
                  set(hObj(12),'CData',LGi);
                  set(hObj(15),'Value',i);

set(hObj(15),'Max',aviObj.NumberOfFrames,'Min',1);
                  CorvisFunction(3);
                  if break_==1
                      break_=0;
                      break
                  end
                  pause(0.01)
              end
          else
              FileName(end-2:end)
              disp('Please select AVI or JPG')
          end
end
if sw==9
  break_=1;
end
if sw==10 % >>>>>>>>>>>>>>>>>>>>>>>>>
          if strcmp(FileName(end-
2:end),'jpg')|strcmp(FileName(end-2:end),'JPG')
              for i=round(get(hObj(15),'Value')):139
                  str = sprintf('%03d',i);
                  LGi=imread([PathName,FileName(1:end-
7),str,FileName(end-3:end)]);
```

```
                              LGi=double(LGi)/255;
                              set(hObj(12),'CData',LGi);
                              set(hObj(15),'Value',i);
                              set(hObj(15),'Max',139,'Min',0);
                              CorvisFunction(3);
                              if break_==1
                                  break_=0;
                                  break
                              end
                              pause(0.01)

                    end
              elseif strcmp(FileName(end-2:end),'avi')
                    aviObj = mmreader([PathName,FileName]);
                    for
i=round(get(hObj(15),'Value')):aviObj.NumberOfFrames
                        LGi = read(aviObj, i);
                        LGi=double(LGi(:,:,1))/255;
                        set(hObj(12),'CData',LGi);
                        set(hObj(15),'Value',i);

set(hObj(15),'Max',aviObj.NumberOfFrames,'Min',1);
                        CorvisFunction(3);
                        if break_==1
                            break_=0;
                            break
                        end
                        pause(0.01)
                    end
              else
                    FileName(end-2:end)
                    disp('Please select AVI or JPG')
              end
        end
```

The third and last discussed m-file, namely *CorvisCalcPre*, is related to performing calculations in the image L_G. The order of operations is directly related to the block diagram—Fig. 2.9. When a given operation is not performed, the variable

value is equal to zero, e.g.: *h1 = 0*. Details of the source code of *CorvisCalcPre* are
shown below:

```
function
[LMED,LRM,LQ,LC]=CorvisCalcPre(LG,h1,Norm,Hist,MSE1)
%%%%%%%%%%%%%%%%%%%%%%%%%%%%%%%%%%%%%%%%%
if h1==0
    LMED=LG;
else

    LMED=medfilt2(LG,[h1 h1],'symmetric');
end
%%%%%%%%%%%%%%%%%%%%%%%%%%%%%%%%%%%%%%%%%
if Norm==0 % None
    LRM=LMED;
end
if Norm==1 % LOCAL
    LRM=mat2gray(LMED);
end
if Norm==2 % global
    LRM=zeros(size(LMED));
    for n=1:size(LMED,2)
        LRM(:,n)=mat2gray(LMED(:,n));
    end
end
%%%%%%%%%%%%%%%%%%%%%%%%%%%%%%%%%%%%%%%%%
if Hist==0 % None
    LQ=LRM;
else % Hist
    LQ=histeq(LRM);
end
%%%%%%%%%%%%%%%%%%%%%%%%%%%%%%%%%%%%%%%%%
if MSE1==0
    LC=LQ;
else
    SE1=ones([MSE1 MSE1]);
    LO=imopen(LQ,SE1);
    LC=abs(LQ-LO);
end
```

Individual actions are intuitive and an interested reader can easily trace them by
analysing the successive lines of the presented source code.

Consequently, the results obtained from the three discussed functions,
CorvisGUI.m, CorvisFunctions.m and *CorvisCalcPre.m*, form the basis for further
analysis, in particular, the image L_C and the source image L_G resulting from image
pre-processing. Details of further analysis are discussed in the next chapter.

Chapter 3
Main Image Processing

3.1 The Known Edge Detection Methods

The methodological and theoretical grounds of edge detection are discussed in detail in the introduction. However, the described theory differs considerably from its practical application. These differences are discussed in this subchapter.

Edge detection is necessary during the analysis of images from the Corvis tonometer for three reasons:

- analysis of the inner and outer edges of the cornea is necessary to determine the pachymetry—corneal thickness,
- analysis of the outer edge of the cornea is necessary to determine the number of biomechanical characteristics of the cornea,
- analysis of the outer edge of the cornea is necessary for texture analysis of the cornea.

Typical edge detection methods can be implemented using one or a combination of several selected functions *edge, filter2* or *conv2*. The first function, with parameters directly defining the type of detector: Sobel, Prewitt or Canny, is the one which is most commonly used. The obtained results for the three listed types of edge detectors, images L_{DS}, L_{DP}, L_{DC} respectively, are shown directly in images L_G by converting pixels to white in places where edges occur (images L_{DSG}, L_{DPG}, L_{DCG} respectively), i.e.:

© Springer International Publishing Switzerland 2016
R. Koprowski, *Image Analysis for Ophthalmological Diagnosis*,
Studies in Computational Intelligence 631, DOI 10.1007/978-3-319-29546-6_3

```
cd('C:/data');

[FileName,PathName] = uigetfile('*.jpg','Select the
Corvis JPG file');
i=70;
str = sprintf('%03d',i);
LG=imread([PathName,FileName(1:end-
7),str,FileName(end-3:end)]);
LG=double(LG)/255;
LDS=edge(LG,'Sobel');
LDP=edge(LG,'Prewitt');
LDC=edge(LG,'Canny',0.2,0.99);
LDSG=LG; LDSG(LDS==1)=1;
LDPG=LG; LDPG(LDP==1)=1;
LDCG=LG; LDCG(LDC==1)=1;
figure; imshow(LDSG);
xlabel('n [pix-
el]','FontSize',20,'FontAngle','Italic');
ylabel('m [pix-
el]','FontSize',20,'FontAngle','Italic');
figure; imshow(LDPG);
xlabel('n [pix-
el]','FontSize',20,'FontAngle','Italic');
ylabel('m [pix-
el]','FontSize',20,'FontAngle','Italic');
figure; imshow(LDCG);
xlabel('n [pix-
el]','FontSize',20,'FontAngle','Italic');
ylabel('m [pix-
el]','FontSize',20,'FontAngle','Italic');
```

The results are shown in Fig. 3.1.

The presented results show that the Canny edge detector is the best. Unfortunately, even this type of detector has drawbacks which include:

- lack of edge continuity,
- a significant amount of noise in the form of isolated white pixels as well as pixels forming small groups—several, several dozen,
- no possibility of medical interpretation of detected edges.

For these reasons, especially the last one, new corneal edge detection methods will be proposed.

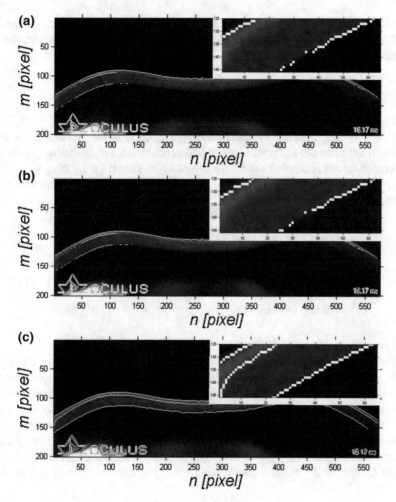

Fig. 3.1 Images L_{DSG}, L_{DPG}, L_{DCG} and their zooms in the range $m \in (1, 65)$, $n \in (125, 146)$ obtained from the image L_G by converting pixels to white in places where edges were detected, images **a** L_{DS}, **b** L_{DP}, **c** L_{DC} respectively

3.2   The First New Edge Detection Method

The need to propose new, dedicated, corneal edge detection methods is due mainly to the need to ensure its continuity and diagnostic interpretation. In this case, the discussed method was initially limited to the detection of the outer corneal edge. At the outset, it can be assumed that for each column of the image $L_G(m, n)$ there is at most one point of the outer corneal edge $L_d(n)$. In the absence of the corneal contour, the obtained values will be equal to M. After a rough analysis of the results obtained during image pre-processing, it turned out that one of the methods that can provide satisfactory results is looking for the greatest gradient in relation to specific points of the selected column in the image L_G, L_{MED} or L_O. For example, for the image L_G it will be $L_{dG}(n)$ equal to:

$$L_{dG}(n) = \arg\max_m (L_G(m,n) - L_G(m+1,n)) \tag{3.1}$$

$m \in (1, M - 1)$.

If there is more than one identical maximum value, only the first one in the order in which the rows are analysed is taken into account. This is due to the position of the cornea which is the first object when looking at the image L_G from the top. At this point, I encourage readers to test the following source code fragment (after having loaded the image L_G):

```
Ld=ones([1 size(LG,2)])*size(LG,2);
LDU=LG;
for n=1:size(LG,2)
    m_ = find(diff(LG(:,n))==max(diff(LG(:,n))));
    Ld(n)=m_(1);
    LDU(m_(1),n)=1;
end
```

The proposed method has its drawbacks. The main ones are high sensitivity to noise and brighter objects that occur in the depth of the eye, for example, parts of the iris which are often visible. A similar situation takes place after the removal of uneven background or histogram equalization. Therefore, it is necessary to carry out additional methods which will later allow for unambiguous determination of the outer corneal contour. These methods include morphological methods, in particular, erosion and dilation. In the case of a symmetrical structural element SE_2, a new image L_C will be determined after a close operation with the following formula:

$$L_C(m,n) = \min_{m,n \in SE_2} \left(\max_{m,n \in SE_2} (L_{MED}(m,n)) \right) \tag{3.2}$$

An important element is the size of the structural element SE_2. This size has been tested in the range from $M_{SE2} \times N_{SE2} = 3 \times 3$ pixels to $M_{SE2} \times N_{SE2} = 13 \times 13$ pixels. This will be further a parameter set by the application user. The next step, directly related to morphological opening, is automatic histogram analysis—L_{HIST}. The designated histogram is subjected to careful analysis. For the counted number of pixels, for example, for the image L_{MED}:

$$L_B(m,n,p_{r2}) = \begin{cases} 1 & \text{if } L_{MED}(m,n) = p_{r2} \\ 0 & \text{other} \end{cases} \tag{3.3}$$

$$L_{HIST}(p_{r2}) = \sum_{n=1}^{N} \sum_{m=1}^{M} L_B(m, n, p_{r2}) \tag{3.4}$$

where $L_{HIST}(p_{r2})$ contains a number of brightness pixels equal to the value p_{r2}. In the next step, the binary image L_{BIN1} is obtained, i.e.:

$$L_{BIN1}(m, n) = \begin{cases} 1 & \text{if } L_{MED}(m, n) \geq \dfrac{\left(\max\limits_{p_{r2}}(L_{HIST}(p_{r2})) \right)}{p_{r3}} \\ 0 & \text{other} \end{cases} \tag{3.5}$$

where p_{r3} is the threshold selected once during the analysis, $p_{r3} \in (2, 20)$. These relationships can be easily written as a code in the following form:

```
cd('C:/data');
[FileName,PathName] = uigetfile('*.jpg','Select the
Corvis JPG file');
figure;
i=72;
str = sprintf('%03d',i);
LG=imread([PathName,FileName(1:end-
7),str,FileName(end-3:end)]);
LMED=medfilt2(LG,[3 11]);
for pr3=2:5:17
    LC=imclose(LMED,ones([3 3]));
    pr2=0:255;
    LHIST= hist(double(LC(:)),pr2);
    pr2LHIST=[pr2',LHIST'];
    pr2LHIST(pr2LHIST(:,2)<(max(LHIST)/pr3),:)=[];
    LBIN=LMED>pr2LHIST(end,1);
    figure
    bar(pr2',LHIST'); grid on; hold on
    line([0 255],[(max(LHIST)/pr3)
(max(LHIST)/pr3)],'LineWidth',5)
    xlabel('L_{HIST}(p_{r2})
[/]','FontSize',20,'FontAngle','Italic');
    ylabel('p_{r2}
[pixel]','FontSize',20,'FontAngle','Italic');
    figure
    imshow(LBIN);
    xlabel('n
[pixel]','FontSize',20,'FontAngle','Italic');
    ylabel('m
[pixel]','FontSize',20,'FontAngle','Italic');
end
```

The above code includes new functions such as: *hist* designed to calculate the histogram for brightness values in the range (0.255), and *bar* and *line* associated with the GUI and providing a bar graph and a line. In the above code, the value p_{r3} was changed in the range $p_{r3} \in (2, 7, 12, 17)$. The results obtained for $i = 72$ and $p_{r3} = 2$ as well as $p_{r3} = 7$ are shown in Fig. 3.2.

The images L_{BIN} shown in Fig. 3.2 enable, at this stage, to determine the correct position of the outer corneal contour. However, the fact that the cornea is the largest object on the scene allows for the use of another operation—labelling. Labelling enables to replace the successive values of clusters in the binary image with their labels. The function *bwlabel* is designed for this purpose. Assuming that two

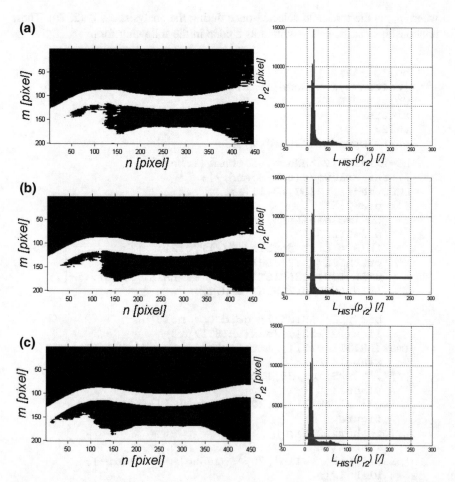

Fig. 3.2 Image L_{BIN} and histogram of the image L_{MED} for $i = 72$ and $p_{r3} = 2$ (**a**); $p_{r3} = 7$ (**b**) and $p_{r3} = 17$ (**c**). Additionally, the histogram graphs show in blue the cut-off line, the thresholding line

vectors, the label and the area corresponding to its cluster, will be stored in the variable *pam*, this fragment of the source code can be written as:

```
LLAB=bwlabel(LBIN);
pam=[];
for lab=1:max(LLAB)
    pam=[pam;[lab sum(sum(LLAB==lab))]];
end
pam_s=sortrows(pam,-2);
LBIN2=LLAB==pam_s(1,1);
```

This method is applicable in all situations for which the object of interest is the largest of all objects and there is a significant amount of noise. As shown in Fig. 3.3, all isolated small objects visible on the right side of the image have been removed. Unfortunately, the shape of the largest object, the cornea, remains unchanged after this operation. In this case, distortions of the outer corneal contour are visible—mainly in the right part of the image (Fig. 3.3).

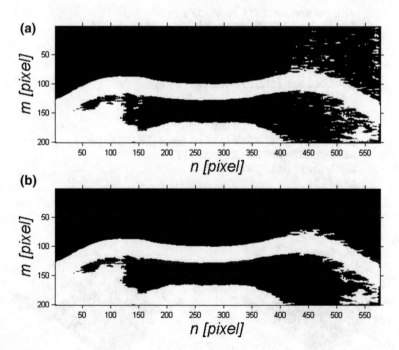

Fig. 3.3 Image L_{BIN} (**a**), and binary image L_{BIN2} (**b**) with only the largest object left

However, the binary image L_{BIN2}, owing to the automatic adjustment of the binarization threshold (Fig. 3.2), provides correct analysis results. Using a simple method for finding the first value equal to one in each column of the image, it is possible to find the waveform of the outer contour $L_{dBIN2}(n)$ with no significant obstacles:

$$L_{dBIN2}(n) = \arg \min_m (L_{BIN2}(m,n)) \qquad (3.6)$$

for $L_{BIN2}(m, n) = 1$.

This method, used for i images, enables to obtain a three-dimensional image, the outer surface, the reaction of the eyeball to an air puff—the waveform $L_E(n, i)$—Fig. 3.4.

The source code providing the image $L_E(n, i)$ is shown below:

```
cd('C:/data');
[FileName,PathName] = uigetfile('*.jpg','Select the
Corvis JPG file');
figure; LE=[];hObj = waitbar(0,'Please wait...');
for i=0:139;
    str = sprintf('%03d',i);
    LG=imread([PathName,FileName(1:end-
7),str,FileName(end-3:end)]);
    LMED=medfilt2(LG,[3 11]);
    pr3=2;
    LC=imclose(LMED,ones([3 3]));
    pr2=0:255;
    LHIST= hist(double(LC(:)),pr2);
    pr2LHIST=[pr2',LHIST'];
    pr2LHIST(pr2LHIST(:,2)<(max(LHIST)/pr3),:)=[];
    LBIN=LMED>pr2LHIST(end,1);
    LLAB=bwlabel(LBIN);
    pam=[];
```

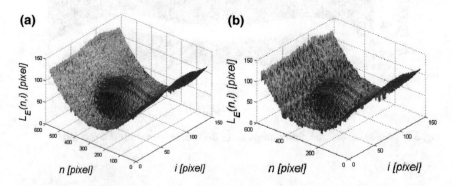

Fig. 3.4 Image $L_E(n, i)$ obtained for **a** $p_{r3} = 10$ and **b** $p_{r3} = 2$

```
      for lab=1:max(LLAB)
          pam=[pam;[lab sum(sum(LLAB==lab))]];

      end
      pam_s=sortrows(pam,-2);
      LBIN2=LLAB==pam_s(1,1);
      [n,m]=meshgrid(1:size(LBIN2,2),1:size(LBIN2,1));
      Ln=n.*LBIN2; Ln(Ln==0)=size(LBIN2,2)+1;
      Lm=m.*LBIN2; Lm(Lm==0)=size(LBIN2,1)+1;
      LE(1:size(Lm,2),i+1)=min(Lm);
      waitbar(i/139,hObj)
end
close(hObj)
figure
surfl(LE); grid on
xlabel('i
[pixel]','FontSize',20,'FontAngle','Italic');
ylabel('n
[pixel]','FontSize',20,'FontAngle','Italic');
zlabel('L_E(n,i)
[pixel]','FontSize',20,'FontAngle','Italic');
shading interp
colormap gray
view(-50,42)
```

It is possible to eliminate small artefacts and noise in the image $L_E(n, i)$ (Fig. 3.4), for example, by applying a median filter or by using the time correction of the edge position which is described below.

3.3   The Second New Edge Detection Method

The second edge detection method, independent of the first one, is based on the results obtained from the Canny detector. The assumption that for each column of the image $L_G(m, n)$ there is at most one point of the outer corneal edge $L_d(n)$ is of great importance here. The image L_{DC} with edges detected with the Canny method (Fig. 3.1) will be used here as well. The sought outer corneal contour will ideally be the first contour in the matrix of the image L_{DC}. In practice, only some of the images satisfy this assumption. Therefore, the method of polynomial curve fitting has been proposed—Fig. 3.5.

Figure 3.5 shows a portion of the cornea seen as grey pixels and the edge detected by the Canny method and marked with black bold edges of the object pixels. The visible object edge was divided into three clusters ($L_{DC}^{(1)}$, $L_{DC}^{(2)}$, $L_{DC}^{(3)}$—the superscript denotes the number of cluster), marked with consecutive

Fig. 3.5 Portion of an object (the cornea) with a contour marked using the Canny method L_{DC} and polynomial curve fitting to cluster pairs

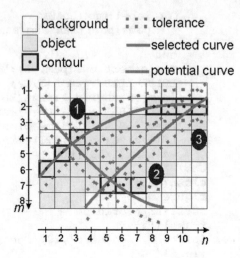

Table 3.1 Total number of pixels located in the tolerance range of ±1 pixel for different configurations of cluster pairs

Cluster	1	2	3
1	4	4	8
2	4	3	3
3	8	3	4

numbers in the black background. The criterion for the division into clusters refers to the maximum possible difference between adjacent pixels in the row axis. In this case, it was a difference of 4 and 5 pixels. Each possible pair, as well as each individual cluster, participates in polynomial curve fitting (red solid lines and one green solid line—Fig. 3.5). For each fitted polynomial curve, contour pixels are counted in a pre-set tolerance range, for example $p_{r4} = \pm 1$ pixel (curves marked with dashed lines). The results obtained for the case presented in Fig. 3.5 are shown in Table 3.1. The sum of pixels presented in Table 3.1 refers to pixels counted within the adopted tolerance range of ±1 pixel for each pair of clusters of the contour portion. It was assumed that a pixel is in the afore-mentioned tolerance range if the coordinates of its centre (indicated by a black point in Fig. 3.5) are within this range. The results in Table 3.1 clearly indicate that the best polynomial curve fitting is for the cluster pairs 1 and 3. The polynomial curve will, in practice, be determined for all i images of the cornea and will be hereinafter referred to as $L_F(n, i)$. The source code enabling to perform the above calculations fully automatically is presented below.

```
cd('C:/data');
[FileName,PathName] = uigetfile('*.jpg','Select the
Corvis JPG file');
pr4=2; pr5=10; pr6=8; LF=[];hObj = waitbar(0,'Please
wait...');
for i=0:139;
    str = sprintf('%03d',i);
    LG=imread([PathName,FileName(1:end-
7),str,FileName(end-3:end)]);
    LG=double(LG)/255;
    LDC=edge(LG,'Canny',0.2,0.99);
    [n,m]=meshgrid(1:size(LDC,2),1:size(LDC,1));
    Ln=n.*LDC; Ln(Ln==0)=size(LDC,2)+1;
    Lm=m.*LDC; Lm(Lm==0)=size(LDC,1)+1;
    LFi=min(Lm);
    LFis=bwlabel(abs([diff(LFi) 0])<pr4);
    pam2=[];
    if max(LFis(:))>0
    for id1=1:max(LFis(:))
        for id2=id1:max(LFis(:))
            LFist=(LFis==id1)|(LFis==id2);
            n=1:length(LFi);
            n(LFist==0)=[]; LFi_=LFi;
            LFi_(LFist==0)=[];
            p = polyfit(n,LFi_,pr6);
            y = polyval(p,1:length(LFi));
            pam2=[pam2;[id1 id2 sum( abs(LFi-y)<pr5
)]];
        end
    end
    end
    pam3=sortrows(pam2,-3);
    LFist=(LFis==pam3(1,1))|(LFis==pam3(1,2));
    n=1:length(LFi);
    n(LFist==0)=[]; LFi_=LFi;
    LFi_(LFist==0)=[];
    p = polyfit(n,LFi_,pr6);
    LF(1:length(LFi),i+1) = polyval(p,1:length(LFi));
    waitbar(i/139,hObj)
end
close(hObj)
figure
surfl(LF); grid on
xlabel('i [pix-
el]','FontSize',20,'FontAngle','Italic');
    ylabel('n [pix-
    el]','FontSize',20,'FontAngle','Italic');
    zlabel('L_F(n,i) [pix-
    el]','FontSize',20,'FontAngle','Italic');
    shading interp
    colormap gray
    view(-50,42)
```

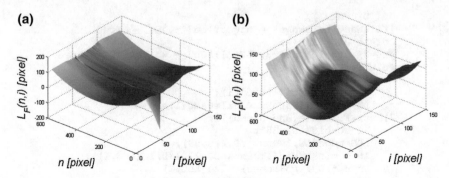

Fig. 3.6 Image $L_F(n, i)$ obtained for **a** $p_{r6} = 3$ and **b** $p_{r6} = 8$

The above source code includes the function *sortrows* which is designed to sort the rows with respect to a given column. Polynomial curve fitting was carried out using the functions *polyfit* and *polyval*. The variables which were set once for all the analysed images included the threshold responsible for the division of the contour into clusters, $p_{r4} = \pm 2$ pixels, and the tolerance threshold with respect to which the contour points are counted, $p_{r5} = \pm 10$ pixels (see Fig. 3.5). The degree of the polynomial p_{r6} was set at 8 taking into account the anthropometric data. Other (mainly lower) polynomial degrees give incorrect results. Figure 3.6 shows two different results for different values of the polynomial degree.

At this point, I encourage readers to test the effect of different values of the thresholds p_{r4}, p_{r5} and the polynomial degree p_{r6} on the obtained results.

3.4   The Third New Edge Detection Method

The image analysis and processing methods discussed in the two previous sub-chapters are based on the analysis of single, independent 2D images. This sub-chapter presents a method based on the analysis of a 3D image. The basis here is the matrix $L_{GA}(n, i, m)$ formed from a sequence of images $L_G(m, n)$. The order of variables in the matrix L_{GA} was changed deliberately because of the reference to the nomenclature in the previous chapters where columns come first and then there are i images. The use of the function *smooth3* enables to filter the image in 3D space and other functions directly responsible for visualization, *patch, isosurface*, or functions responsible for lighting, *camlight, lighting phong*. The results are shown in Fig. 3.7.

Figure 3.7 also shows the image $L_{GAS}(n, i, m)$ resulting from 3D filtration of the image $L_{GA}(n, i, m)$ with the use of the mask h_3 sized $M_{h3} \times N_{h3} \times I_{h3} = 7 \times 7 \times 7$ pixels. The basis is the matrix $L_{GA}(n, i, m)$ created by using the following source code:

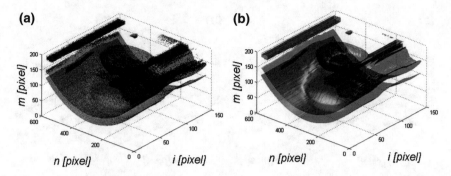

Fig. 3.7 Image $L_{GA}(n, i, m)$ (**a**) and the image $L_{GAS}(n, i, m)$ resulting from 3D filtration of the image $L_{GA}(n, i, m)$ with the use of the mask h_3 sized $M_{h3} \times N_{h3} \times I_{h3} = 7 \times 7 \times 7$ pixels

```
cd('C:/data');
[FileName,PathName] = uigetfile('*.jpg','Select the
Corvis JPG file');
LGA=[]; LH=[]; pr7=0.1; hObj = waitbar(0,'Please
wait...');
for i=0:139;
    str = sprintf('%03d',i);
    LG=imread([PathName,FileName(1:end-
7),str,FileName(end-3:end)]);
    LG=double(LG)/255;
    LGA(1:size(LG,2),i+1,1:size(LG,1))=LG';
    waitbar(i/139,hObj)
end
close(hObj)
```

The created matrix $L_{GA}(n, i, m)$ occupies 129,024,000 bytes in the Matlab workspace. Raster (variables n, m, i), necessary to create the graphs shown in Fig. 3.7 is of exactly the same size, i.e.:

```
[n,m,i]=meshgrid(1:size(LGA,2),1:size(LGA,1),1:size
(LGA,3))
```

Filtration was performed using the function *smooth3*, i.e.:

```
LGAS=smooth3(LGA,'box',7);
```

The next step involved separation of the outer corneal contour from the image $L_{GAS}(n, i, m)$. The method is similar to the fragment of the second method presented in the previous subchapter in which the first white pixels of a binary image are found for each of the columns. Using the following source code (the subsequent processing steps):

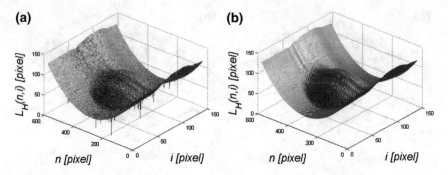

Fig. 3.8 Image $L_H(n, i)$ obtained from the image $L_{GA}(n, i, m)$ **a** without filtration and the image $L_H(n, i)$ resulting from 3D filtration of the image $L_{GA}(n, i, m)$ with the use of the mask h_3 sized $M_{h3} \times N_{h3} \times I_{h3} = 3 \times 3 \times 3$ pixels ($L_{GAS}(n, i, m)$)

```
LH=[];
for i=0:139
    [n,m]=meshgrid(1:size(LGAS,1),1:size(LGAS,3));
    LBIN=[];
    LBIN(1:576,1:200)=LGAS(:,i+1,:)>pr7; LBIN=LBIN';
    Lm=m.*LBIN; Lm(Lm==0)=size(LBIN,1)+1;
    LH(1:size(Lm,2),i+1)=min(Lm);
end
```

two different results presented in Fig. 3.8 were obtained. They come from the analysis of the images $L_{GA}(n, i, m)$ and $L_{GAS}(n, i, m)$ with the use of the mask h_3 sized $M_{h3} \times N_{h3} \times I_{h3} = 3 \times 3 \times 3$ pixels.

The image $L_H(n, i)$ without 3D filtration includes numerous small incorrect locations of pixels—it is best seen in Fig. 3.8 a. The image $L_H(n, i)$ after filtration using the mask h_3 sized $M_{h3} \times N_{h3} \times I_{h3} = 3 \times 3 \times 3$ pixels is the result of the presented third approach to edge detection.

The next subchapter presents a comparison of the three methods of corneal edge detection in an image sequence which are described above.

3.5   Comparison of the Three New Methods of Corneal Edge Detection

The previous chapters presented three independent methods for detecting the outer contour of the cornea. They resulted in the following images:

$L_E(n, i)$ approach based on binarization with an automatically selected threshold of 2D images,

$L_F(n, i)$ approach based on approximation of the edge detected with the Canny method using a polynomial for single 2D images,

$L_H(n, i)$ approach based on 3D reconstruction.

These methods will be compared on the basis of the same sequence of 2D images. The first part will involve the comparison of the accuracy of contour detection.

When tracing the anthropometric data and the maximum corneal deformation, it can be observed that the difference in the position of the corneal edge for subsequent columns (variable n) does not exceed 2 pixels. All the major differences in adjacent pixels of the corneal edge can therefore be considered noise. Additionally, the images $L_E(n, i)$, $L_F(n, i)$ and $L_H(n, i)$ were compared with the image $L_R(n, i)$ obtained from the manual analysis of the contour waveform in individual 2D images. $L_R(n, i)$ was determined by an expert and is further treated as a reference image. The results obtained are shown in Fig. 3.9.

The formulas (1.16) and (1.17) for the adopted threshold $p_{r8} \in (1, 4)$, discussed in the introduction, were used for further analysis of errors. The results obtained are shown in Table 3.2.

The results presented in Table 3.2 clearly indicate that the first method has the highest error value (78, 25.5 %, depending on the adopted value of the threshold). Relatively large differences are also apparent for the first method in Fig. 3.9. The second method has the smallest error value, but the possibility of incorrect contour approximation using the described polynomial should be taken into account. This may result in very large discrepancies between the actual contour and the one determined with this method. From a practical point of view, the third method

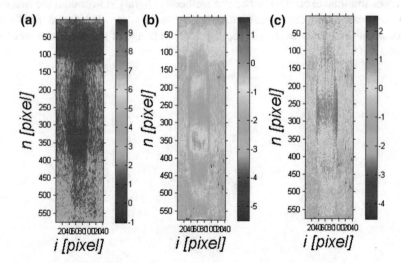

Fig. 3.9 Image of the difference values expressed in pixels: between images $L_R(n, i)$ and $L_E(n, i)$—graph (**a**), between $L_R(n, i)$ and $L_F(n, i)$—graph (**b**), between $L_R(n, i)$ and $L_H(n, i)$—graph (**c**)

Table 3.2 Values of the measurement error δ_g for different values of the threshold $p_{r8} \in (1, 4)$

Value of threshold p_{r8}	Method		
	First $L_E(n, i)$ [%]	Second $L_F(n, i)$ [%]	Third $L_H(n, i)$ [%]
1 pixel	78	0.06	3.09
2 pixels	25.5	0	0.03
3 pixels	7.3	0	0
4 pixels	2.1	0	0

Table 3.3 Time of calculating contour images $L_E(n, i)$, $L_F(n, i)$ and $L_H(n, i)$ for Intel Xenon X5680 3.33 GHz

Method		
First—$L_E(n, i)$	Second—$L_F(n, i)$	Third—$L_H(n, i)$
3.14 s	9.27 s	5.33 s

seems to be the best. It does not use polynomial approximation and is significantly more precise in comparison with the first method.

Measurement of computation time was performed without visualization of the results by providing the access path. The results for Intel Xenon processor X5680 3.33 GHz and Windows 7, Matlab Version 7.11.0.584 (R2010b) are shown in Table 3.3.

As is apparent from Table 3.3, the first method provides results the fastest. However, due to a fairly high error of this method, it can be considered as a preliminary method for approximate analyses. The second method is the slowest, computation time exceeds 9 s. The last method is slightly slower than the first one. For this reason and due to the smallest error values, it will be used for further calculations and analyses. It will be, therefore, an image of the outer contour of the cornea $L_H(n, i)$.

Chapter 4
Additional Image Processing and Measurement

Modern methods of image analysis and processing allow not only for the automatic separation of the corneal contour but also for analyses which are biomechanically and medically interesting. The image of the outer corneal contour $L_H(n, i)$ and the image of the cornea $L_G(m, n, i)$ in a sequence, whose method of obtaining is presented in the previous chapter, are fundamental to this type of analysis. The features obtained on this basis, which are diagnostically important parameters, are in the following subchapters marked with the symbol w. The first one is texture analysis of the cornea.

4.1 Texture Analysis of the Cornea

Texture analysis is a fully-developed part of the image analysis and processing methods. Most texture analysis methods are based on statistics and ROI analysis. In the present case, the behaviour of the cornea, and to be more exact, the behaviour of its texture during deformation is of interest. In the first stage of analysis, the cornea needs to be separated from a sequence of images $L_G(m, n, i)$. For this purpose, a constant value of corneal thickness is assumed (which is justified only within certain limits) that is further referred to as $p_{r9} = 20$ pixels. The image of the cornea texture for all i images $L_{GK}(m_i, n)$ will be therefore equal to:

$$L_{GK}(m_i, n) = L_G(m, n, i) \qquad (4.1)$$

for $m \in (L_K(n, i), L_K(n, i) + p_{r9})$ and $m_i \in (1, p_{r9})$.

The image $L_{GK}(m_i, n)$ is shown in Fig. 4.1.

Figure 4.1 shows the corneal texture separated from individual i images $L_G(m, n)$ for the adopted constant thickness $p_{r9} = 20$ pixels. Local shifts of recurrent elements of the corneal texture are visible in Fig. 4.1. Their further analysis

© Springer International Publishing Switzerland 2016
R. Koprowski, *Image Analysis for Ophthalmological Diagnosis*,
Studies in Computational Intelligence 631, DOI 10.1007/978-3-319-29546-6_4

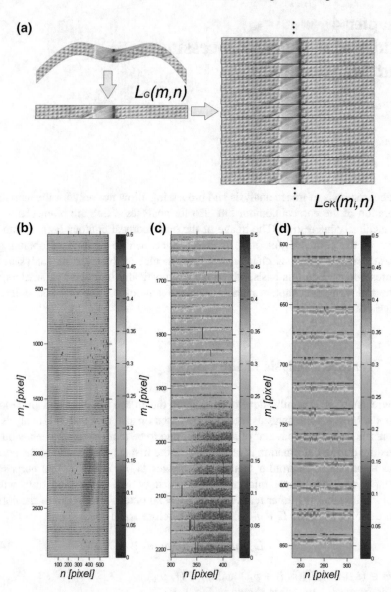

Fig. 4.1 Schematic diagram of rules of corneal texture conversion **a** actual image $L_{GK}(m_i, n)$, **b–d** zoom of its selected fragments

involves the removal of the brightest and darkest rows using double-threshold binarization for which:

$$L_{GKS}(m_i) = \frac{1}{N} \cdot \sum_{n=1}^{N} L_{GK}(m_i, n) \qquad (4.2)$$

$$L_{BIN3}(m_i) = \begin{cases} 1 & if & L_{GKS}(m_i) > (L_{GKSM}(m_i) - p_{r10}) \wedge \\ & & L_{GKS}(m_i) < (L_{GKSM}(m_i) + p_{r10}) \\ 0 & other \end{cases} \qquad (4.3)$$

where:

$L_{GKSM}(m_i)$ the result of median filtering of $L_{GKS}(m_i)$

p_{r10}—threshold, adopted arbitrarily as 0.001, responsible for the tolerance range during double-threshold binarization, i.e.: $L_{GKSM}(m_i) + p_{r10}$ and $L_{GKSM}(m_i) - p_{r10}$.

The waveform of $L_{BIN3}(m_i)$ has values equal to 0 for the extreme brightness of pixels calculated as the mean value for each row. A new image $L_{GB}(m_k, n)$ is therefore a combination of the selected rows from the image $L_{GK}(m_i, n)$. This selection was indicated by the value "1" in $L_{BIN3}(m_i)$, i.e.:

$$L_{GB}(m_k, n) = L_{GB}(m_i, n) \; if \; L_{BIN3}(m_i) = 1 \qquad (4.4)$$

The source code allowing for the performance of the above calculations as well as the results are shown below (Fig. 4.2).

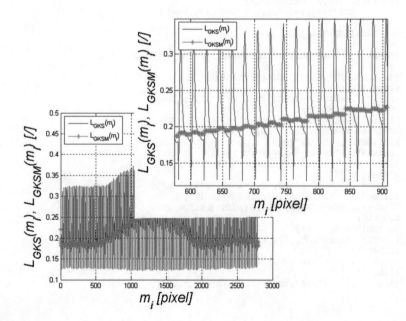

Fig. 4.2 Graph $L_{GKS}(m_i)$—blue, and graph $L_{GKSM}(m_i)$—red, with the zoom of a selected fragment

```
cd('C:/data');
[FileName,PathName] = uigetfile('*.jpg','Select the
Corvis JPG file');
LG=[]; LH=[]; pr7=0.1; pr9=20; pr10=0.001; hObj =
waitbar(0,'Please wait ...');
for i=0:139;
    str = sprintf('%03d',i);
    LGi=imread([PathName,FileName(1:end-
7),str,FileName(end-3:end)]);
    LGi=double(LGi)/255;
    LG(1:size(LGi,2),i+1,1:size(LGi,1))=LGi';
    waitbar(i/139,hObj)
end
close(hObj)
LGS=smooth3(LG,'box',1);

end
close(hObj)
LGS=smooth3(LG,'box',1);
LH=[];
LGK=[];
for i=0:139
    [n,m]=meshgrid(1:size(LGS,1),1:size(LGS,3));
    LBIN=[];

LBIN(1:size(LGS,1),1:size(LGS,3))=LGS(:,i+1,:)>pr7;
    LBIN=LBIN';
    Lm=m.*LBIN; Lm(Lm==0)=size(LBIN,1)+1;
    Lmm=round(min(Lm));
    LH(1:size(Lm,2),i+1)=Lmm;
    LGK_=[];
    for n=1:size(Lm,2)
        Lp=Lmm(n);
        Lk=(Lmm(n)+pr9-1);
Lk(Lk>size(Lm,1))=size(Lm,1);
        LGK_(1:(Lk-Lp+1),n)=LGS(n,i+1,Lp:Lk);
    end
    LGK=[LGK;LGK_];
end
figure; imshow(LGK,[]); colormap([jet(256);jet(256)]);
xlabel('n
[pixel]','FontSize',20,'FontAngle','Italic');
ylabel('m_{i}
[pixel]','FontSize',20,'FontAngle','Italic');
LGKS=mean(LGK',1);
figure; plot(LGKS); hold on
LGKSM=medfilt2(LGKS,[1 19],'symmetric');
plot(LGKSM,'-r*'); grid on
ylabel('L_{GKS}(m_i), L_{GKSM}(m_i)
[/]','FontSize',20,'FontAngle','Italic');
xlabel('m_{i}
[pixel]','FontSize',20,'FontAngle','Italic');
legend('L_{GKS}(m_i)', 'L_{GKSM}(m_i)')
LBIN3=((LGKS<(LGKSM+pr10))&(LGKS>(LGKSM-pr10)))';
LGB=LGK;
LGB(LBIN3==0,:)=[];
figure; imshow(LGB,[]); colormap('jet')
xlabel('n
[pixel]','FontSize',20,'FontAngle','Italic');
ylabel('m_{k}
[pixel]','FontSize',20,'FontAngle','Italic');
```

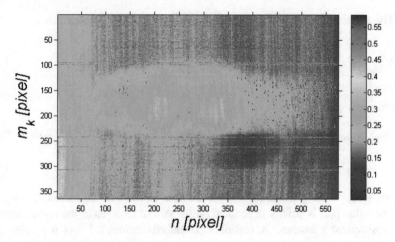

Fig. 4.3 Image $L_{GB}(m_k, n)$

The resulting image $L_{GB}(m_k, n)$ is shown in Fig. 4.3.

The graph $L_{GKS}(m_i)$ is the characteristic of the corneal texture both because of the contrast between the brightness values (minimum and maximum—Fig. 4.2) and the reproducibility obtainable for subsequent i images of the cornea. At this point, I encourage readers to trace the results obtained for $L_{GKS}(m_i) < L_{GKSM}(m_i)$ and $L_{GKS}(m_i) > L_{GKSM}(m_i)$. The removal of extreme brightness values in the described case provides the image $L_{GB}(m_k, n)$ (Fig. 4.3) and enables to trace the brightness changes for successive values of m_k. As shown in the illustrated image $L_{GB}(m_k, n)$, there is a shift of typical texture fragments. The use of the Grey Level Co-occurrence Matrix (GLCM) provides information about local texture shifts during corneal deformation. The idea of using GLCM to evaluate statistical indicators of texture shifts is shown in Fig. 4.4.

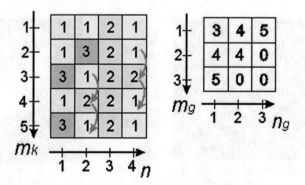

Fig. 4.4 Schematic diagram of calculating the matrix $L_{GLCM}(m_g, n_g)$ (*right*) based on the sample matrix $L_{GB}(m_k, n)$ (*left*) for $p_{r11} = 1$ in the vertical neighbourhood. Examples of counted vertical neighbourhoods of the values "1" and "2" are marked in *red*

The formal notation of the discussed method GLCM is shown below.

$$L_{GLCM}(m_g, n_g) = \sum_{n=1}^{N} \sum_{m_i=1}^{M_i} L_{GL}(m_i, n, m_g, n_g) \tag{4.5}$$

where:

$$L_{GL}(m_k, n, m_g, n_g) = \begin{cases} 1 & \text{if} & \left(L_{GB}(m_k, n) = m_g\right) \bigwedge \left(L_{GB}(m_k + p_{r11}, n) = n_g\right) \\ 0 & \text{other} \end{cases}$$

$$\tag{4.6}$$

for $m_k + p_{r11} \leq M_{GB}$ where M_{GB} is the number of rows of the matrix $L_{GB}(m_k, n)$.

The value p_{r11} is strictly dependent on the rate of changes in the texture content for subsequent i images. A preliminary analysis confirmed that the value p_{r11} should be absolute and lie in the range $p_{r11} \in (M_{GB}/40 \; M_{GB}/10)$ pixels. The result, namely the image $L_{GLCM}(m_g, n_g)$, for $p_{r11} = M_{GB}/40$ is shown in Fig. 4.5.

These images were obtained by continuing the subsequent phases of the algorithm operation with the notation:

```
LGLCM = graycomatrix(uint8(round(LGB*255)),'Offset',[-
10 0],'NumLevels',256);
figure; imshow(LGLCM,[]); colormap('jet'); colorbar
xlabel('n_{g}
[pixel]','FontSize',20,'FontAngle','Italic');
ylabel('m_{g}
[pixel]','FontSize',20,'FontAngle','Italic');
LBIN4=LGLCM>1;
axis([1 130 1 130])
```

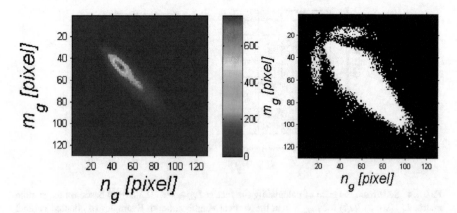

Fig. 4.5 Image $L_{GLCM}(m_g, n_g)$ and its binary image being binarization with a threshold of 1 pixel

Graycomatrix is a function that enables to obtain GLCM transformations. Parameters such as *Offset* allow for precise determination of the inclination angle at which the differences between pixels will be analysed—in this case $p_{r11} = 10$ pixels. Interpretation of the results is intuitive. The distribution of data on the main diagonal of the matrix $L_{GLCM}(m_g, n_g)$ is directly related to the presence of vertical neighbourhoods between pixels of the same or similar brightness. The presence of data in the matrix $L_{GLCM}(m_g, n_g)$ beyond the main diagonal is indicative of differences in brightness of vertically adjacent pixels. Thus, the shape of the distribution of data in the matrix $L_{GLCM}(m_g, n_g)$ resembles an ellipse (especially after binarization—Fig. 4.5). Therefore, quantitative features directly related to changes in the corneal texture are the larger and smaller semi-major axes of the ellipse of the object from the image in Fig. 4.5b. Such measurement can be carried out using the function *regionprop* or *imrotate* in the following notation:

```
LBIN5=imrotate(LBIN4,45,'nearest');
figure; imshow(LBIN5,[]);
dED=sum(sum(LBIN5,1)>0);
dES=sum(sum(LBIN5,2)>0);
```

The results of the size of the larger and smaller semi-major axes are equal in the analysed case, $d_{ED} = 136$, $d_{ES} = 75$ pixels. The main parameter d_{ES} is a quantitative measure of changes in pixel brightness for successive i images, for the area of the cornea. This is the first of the parameters defining quantitatively the eyeball response to an air puff and will be further referred to as $w(1)$, i.e.: $w(1) = d_{ES}$.

4.2 Analysis of the Eyeball Reaction

The outer contour of the cornea sequence $L_H(n, i)$ contains complete information on the response of the eye to an air puff. The contour is made up of three components:

- constant component being the natural shape of the cornea—$L_{HC}(n, i)$,
- eyeball reaction to an air puff—$L_{HO}(n, i)$,
- corneal response to an air puff—$L_{HR}(n, i)$.

Analysis of the eyeball reaction is possible by analysing edges of the image $L_H(n, i)$. They correspond anthropometrically to the sclera fragments. However, the constant component, being the shape of the cornea and sclera fragments, is pre-separated for the initial images during acquisition.

The constant component is the natural shape of the cornea and is visible for the initial images in the sequence. Due to noise present in the image, it is good to average the shape of the cornea for several, several dozen of initial images $L_G(m, n, i)$. On the other hand, the start of the corneal deformation or the eyeball reaction is not precisely known.

The measure of differences is the adopted maximum of the standard deviation of the mean for the image $L_H(n, i)$, i.e.: $L_{STDLH}(i_s)$, measured as:

$$L_{STDLH}(i_s) = \max_{n} \sqrt{\frac{1}{i_s - 1} \sum_{i=1}^{i_s} \left(L_H(n, i) - \frac{1}{i_s} \sum_{i=1}^{i_s} L_H(n, i) \right)^2} \qquad (4.7)$$

In subsequent iterations the value i_s is increased starting from $i_s = 1$. The algorithm stops its work when $L_{STDLH}(i_s) > 1$ or if $i_s = 10$, i.e.:

```
pam=[];
for is=1:size(LH,2)
    pam=[pam;[is, max(std(LH(:,1:is),0,2))]];
end
figure; plot(pam(:,1),pam(:,2),'-g*'); grid on; hold
on
for is=1:10
    if max(std(LH(:,1:is),0,2))>1
        break
    end
    LHC=mean(LH(:,1:is),2)*ones([1 size(LH,2)]);
end
line([is is],[0 max(pam(:,2))],'LineWidth',4)
xlabel('i_s [pix-
el]','FontSize',20,'FontAngle','Italic');
yla-
bel('L_{STDLH}[pixel]','FontSize',20,'FontAngle','Ital
ic');
legend('L_{STDLH}','i_s=p_{r12}')
```

The obtained graph $L_{STDLH}(i_s)$ is shown in Fig. 4.6.

On the basis of the found i_s, the waveform of the constant component $L_{HC}(n, i)$ was calculated, in simple terms independent of i ($L_{HC}(n)$), in the following form:

$$L_{HC}(n) = \frac{1}{i_s} \sum_{i=1}^{i_s} L_H(n, i) \qquad (4.8)$$

The area $i \in (1, i_s)$, from which $L_{HC}(n, i)$ was calculated from the waveform $L_H(n, i)$, is highlighted in red in Fig. 4.7.

Fig. 4.6 Graph $L_{STDLH}(i_s)$ marked in *green* and threshold p_{r12} marked in *blue*

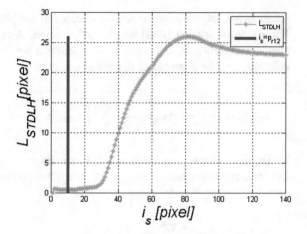

Fig. 4.7 Graph $L_H(n, i)$ (*top*) and $L_{HHC}(n, i)$ (*bottom*). The range $i \in (1, i_s)$ is marked in *red*. The range from $i = 1$ to i_s is marked in *green*

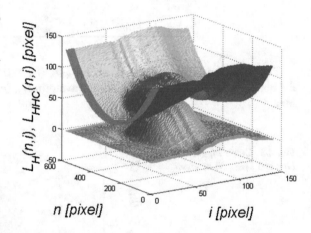

In the next step, using similar methodology, the eyeball reaction was calculated. For this purpose, in a preliminary stage, the waveform $L_{HC}(n, i)$ was subtracted from $L_H(n, i)$ thus obtaining $L_{HHC}(n, i)$, i.e.:

$$L_{HHC}(n, i) = L_H(n, i) - L_{HC}(n, i) \tag{4.9}$$

The waveform $L_{HHC}(n, i)$ is shown in Fig. 4.7 at the bottom. On its basis, the eyeball reaction will be calculated. As already mentioned, information from a sequence of images $L_G(m, n, i)$ on changes in the sclera position on both sides (the extreme columns) of the image will be used here. Since it was assumed that the sclera is not subject to deformation, changes in the position of the eyeball can be linearly reconstructed based on this information. Accordingly, the values of the standard deviation of the mean were calculated for the extreme positions of the columns, i.e., for example to the initial columns:

$$L_{STDLHHC}(n_s) = \max_i \sqrt{\frac{1}{n_s - 1} \sum_{n=1}^{n_s} \left(L_{HHC}(n, i) - \frac{1}{n_s} \sum_{n=1}^{n_s} L_{HHC}(n, i) \right)^2} \quad (4.10)$$

The first value n_s, for which $n_s > 1$, is the sought range $n \in (1, n_s)$. On this basis, the linear reconstruction of changes in the eyeball position is performed—$L_{HO}(n, i)$, i.e.:

$$L_{HO}(n, i) = \frac{1}{n_s} \sum_{n=1}^{n_s} L_{HHC}(n, i)$$
$$+ \frac{\frac{1}{n_s} \sum_{n=1}^{n_s} L_{HHC}(n, i) - \frac{1}{n_s} \sum_{n=N-n_s-1}^{N} L_{HHC}(n, i)}{N} \cdot n \quad (4.11)$$

The characteristic areas of the edges $L_{HHC}(n, i)$ are shown in green in Fig. 4.7 at the bottom. An example of the resulting waveform $L_{HO}(n, i)$ is shown in Fig. 4.8 in blue.

Fig. 4.8 Graph $L_{HO}(n, i)$ in *blue* and $L_{HR}(n, i)$ in *green*

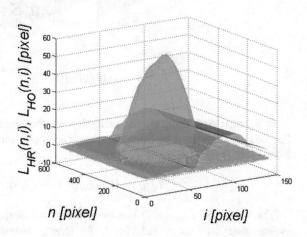

The code of this fragment in Matlab is as follows:

```matlab
LHHC=LH-LHC;
for ns=1:10
    if
(max(std(LHHC(1:ns,:),0,1))>1)|(max(std(LHHC((end-ns-
1):end,:),0,1))>1)
        break
    end
    LP=mean(LHHC(1:ns,:),1);
    LK=mean(LHHC((end-ns-1):end,:),1);
    LHO=[];
    for i=1:length(LP)

LHO(1:size(LHHC,1),i)=linspace(LP(i),LK(i),size(LHHC,1
));
    end
end
figure
hObj1=surfl(LH); grid on; hold on
xlabel('i [pix-
el]','FontSize',20,'FontAngle','Italic');

ylabel('n [pix-
el]','FontSize',20,'FontAngle','Italic');
zlabel('L_H(n,i), L_{HHC}(n,i) [pix-
el]','FontSize',20,'FontAngle','Italic');
hObj2=surfl(LHHC);
view(-34,18)
shading interp
colormap gray
hObj3=surfl(LH(:,1:10));
set(hObj3,'FaceColor','red','EdgeColor','red')
hObj4=surfl(LHHC(1:20,:));
set(hObj4,'FaceColor','green','EdgeColor','green')
[X,Y]=meshgrid(1:size(LHHC((end-
19):end,:),2),1:size(LHHC((end-19):end,:),1));
hObj5=surfl(X,Y+556,LHHC((end-19):end,:));
set(hObj5,'FaceColor','green','EdgeColor','green')
LHR=LHHC-LHO;
figure
hObj6=surfl(LHO); grid on; hold on
set(hObj6,'FaceColor','blue','EdgeColor','none','FaceA
lpha',0.3)
hObj7=surfl(LHR);
set(hObj7,'FaceColor','green','EdgeColor','none','Face
Alpha',0.3)
xlabel('i [pix-
el]','FontSize',20,'FontAngle','Italic');
ylabel('n [pix-
el]','FontSize',20,'FontAngle','Italic');
zlabel('L_{HR}(n,i), L_{HO}(n,i) [pix-
el]','FontSize',20,'FontAngle','Italic');
view(-34,18)
```

The new applied functions include *linspace*. The other functions have already been used before, such as: *hold on* intended to freeze the graph, *grid on* designed to show the rastr in the graph, *surfl* meant to show 3D graphs and their parameters *FaceColor*, *EdgeColor* etc.

On the basis of the waveform of the eyeball reaction $L_{HO}(n, i)$, it is possible to determine a number of useful features in data analysis, for example, for classification.

4.2.1   Distinction Between the Eye Position—Left/Right

Musculi bulbi oculi and the surrounding muscles respond differently to force in the form of an air puff. The eyeball is pushed into the skull. As a consequence, straight and oblique muscles withstand it. Mirror arrangement of these muscles for the left and right eye enables to automatically distinguish between them. This difference is written in the following way using $L_{L/R}$:

$$L_{L/R} = \frac{1}{I} \sum_{i=1}^{I} (L_{HOL}(i) - L_{HOR}(i)) \tag{4.12}$$

where:

$$L_{HOL}(i) = \frac{1}{n_s} \sum_{n=1}^{n_s} L_{HO}(n, i) \tag{4.13}$$

$$L_{HOR}(i) = \frac{1}{n_s} \sum_{n=N-n_s-1}^{N} L_{HO}(n, i) \tag{4.14}$$

Figure 4.9 shows the graph $L_{HOR}(i)$ in red and $L_{HOL}(i)$ in green.

For the verified cases, when $L_{L/R} > 0$, the left eye is analysed and in the other cases ($L_{L/R} < 0$) it is the right eye. The situation when $L_{L/R} = 0$ did not happen during the performed analyses. However, for $L_{L/R} \approx 0$, additional measurements and analyses should be conducted which would confirm whether the left or right eye was analysed. In extreme cases, such situations should be excluded from further analysis. The adequate notation is:

```
LHOL=mean(LHO(1:10,:),1);
LHOR=mean(LHO(end-9:end,:),1);
```

This feature, related to the ability to distinguish between the left and right eye, will also be mentioned in the next subchapter on the occasion of frequency analysis.

Fig. 4.9 Graph $L_{HOR}(i)$ in
red and $L_{HOL}(i)$ in *green*

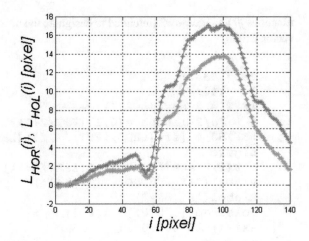

4.2.2   Frequency Analysis

Each of i images was acquired every 231 μs, which gives the acquisition frequency
Fs = 4.33 kHz. Signal recording time is 231 μs * 140 images = 32.340 ms. The
spectrum of the Fourier transform (FFT) L_{FFTHO} is shown in Fig. 4.10 using the

Fig. 4.10 Spectrum L_{FFTHO}
of the waveform $L_{HOR}(i)$ in
red and $L_{HOL}(i)$ in *green*

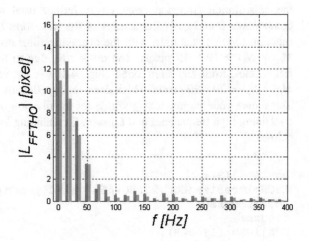

functions *fft* and *nextpow2* (intended to designate the nearest power of 2 of the input vector length):

```
Fs = 4330;
I = 140;
iFFT = 2^nextpow2(I);
f = Fs/2*linspace(0,1,iFFT/2+1);
LFFTHO = [fft(LHOL,iFFT)/I;fft(LHOR,iFFT)/I];
figure
bar(f,2*abs(LFFTHO(:,1:iFFT/2+1))','grouped');
ylabel('|L_{FFTHO}| [pixel]')
xlabel('f [Hz]')
colormap([1 0 0; 0 1 0 ])
axis([-10 400 0 17])
grid on
```

The results obtained are in line with expectations. There is no single dominant harmonic (Fig. 4.10). The spectrum of waveforms $L_{HOR}(i)$ and $L_{HOL}(i)$ may be divided into the range from 0 to 80, 90 Hz for the low frequency components and above 90 Hz for higher frequencies. However, a closer analysis of signals, for example using the Hamming or Blackman window, requires here the use of Matlab toolbox, namely Signal Processing, to which I refer interested readers.

Remaining in the area of the functions available in Image Processing toolbox, the convolution (function *conv2*) was further used to separate low-frequency components from higher frequencies of the waveform $L_{HO}(n, i)$. The convolution function (*conv2*) was used with the averaging filter mask h_5 having a resolution $M_{h5} \times N_{h5} = 19 \times 19$ pixels. The mask size, due to the large separation of low frequencies from the high ones (Fig. 4.10), may vary considerably even to $M_{h5} \times N_{h5} = 29 \times 29$ pixels, which does not significantly affect the results obtained. The source code fragment responsible for the division of $L_{HO}(n, i)$ into $L_{HOH}(n, i)$ containing high frequencies and $L_{HOW}(n, i)$ containing low frequencies is presented below:

```
h5=ones(19);
LHOW=imresize(conv2(LHO,h5,'valid')/sum(h5(:)),size(LHO));
LHOH=LHO-LHOW;
figure;
hObj1=surfl(LHOH);
grid on; hold on
hObj2=surfl(LHOW);
xlabel('i [pixel]','FontSize',20,'FontAngle','Italic');
ylabel('n [pixel]','FontSize',20,'FontAngle','Italic');
zlabel('L_{HOH}(n,i), L_{HOW}(n,i)')
```

```
[pixel]','FontSize',20,'FontAngle','Italic');
shading interp
set(hObj1,'FaceColor',[0 0
0.2],'EdgeColor','none','FaceAlpha',0.3)
set(hObj2,'FaceColor',[0.3 0.3
0.9],'EdgeColor','none','FaceAlpha',0.3)
legend('L_{HOH}(n,i)', 'L_{HOW}(n,i)')
view(-50,42)
LFFTHOH =fft(LHOH(floor(size(LHO,1)/2),:),iFFT)/I;
figure
bar(f,2*abs(LFFTHOH(:,1:iFFT/2+1))','grouped');
ylabel('|L_{FFTHOH}|
[pixel]','FontSize',20,'FontAngle','Italic');
xlabel('f [Hz]','FontSize',20,'FontAngle','Italic');
grid on
axis([0 400 0 1.6])
```

The results obtained are presented in Figs. 4.11 and 4.12.

From a practical point of view (medical practice), scalar values which describe the maximum amplitude of the low and high harmonics as well as the waveforms $L_{HOH}(i)$ and $L_{HOW}(i)$ are vital. These values are further parameters which quantify the eyeball response to force in the form of an air puff, i.e.:

$$w(2) = \max_{n,i} L_{HOW}(n,i) \tag{4.15}$$

$$w(3) = \max_{i} L_{HOW}(1,i) - \max_{i} L_{HOW}(N,i) \tag{4.16}$$

Fig. 4.11 Graph $L_{HOH}(n, i)$ in *black* and $L_{HOW}(n, i)$ in *blue*

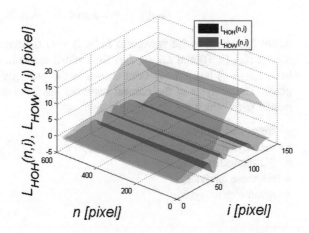

Fig. 4.12 Spectrum L_{FFTHOH} of the waveform $L_{HOH}(i)$

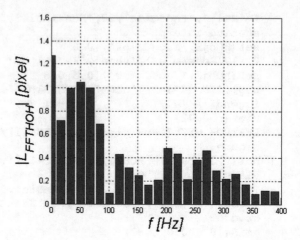

$$w(4) = \max_{n,i} L_{HOH}(n, i) - \min_{n,i} L_{HOH}(n, i) \qquad (4.17)$$

These features will be used further for a comprehensive, quantitative assessment of the eyeball reaction to an air puff from the Corvis tonometer.

4.3   Analysis of the Corneal Response

The corneal response $L_{HR}(n, i)$ is designated based on the information acquired in the previous subchapter, i.e.:

$$L_{HR}(n, i) = L_{HHC}(n, i) - L_{HO}(n, i) \qquad (4.18)$$

where $L_{HHC}(n, i)$ is the waveform $L_H(n, i)$ after the removal of the constant component ($L_{HC}(n, i)$) and $L_{HO}(n, i)$ is the eyeball reaction. An example of the waveform $L_{HR}(n, i)$ has already been shown in the previous subchapter in Fig. 4.8 in green. The analysis of the corneal response has been divided into several fundamental parts which are described below:

- frequency analysis,
- determination of applanation points,
- 3D reconstruction,
- response analysis,
- symmetry analysis.

4.3.1   Frequency Analysis

Frequency analysis of the waveform $L_{HR}(n, i)$ is implemented in an analogous manner to the eyeball response analysis. The division into a low-frequency component $L_{HRW}(n, i)$ from 0 to 90 Hz and $L_{HRH}(n, i)$ above 90 Hz was performed by filtration using an averaging filter with a mask h_6 sized $M_{h6} \times N_{h6} = 19 \times 19$ pixels. The use of the following notation in Matlab resulted in the waveforms $L_{HRH}(n, i)$ and $L_{HRW}(n, i)$: (Fig. 4.13)

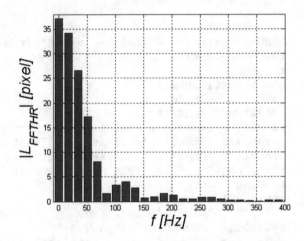

Fig. 4.13 Spectrum L_{FFTHR} of the waveform $L_{HRH}(n, i)$ for n with the highest amplitude

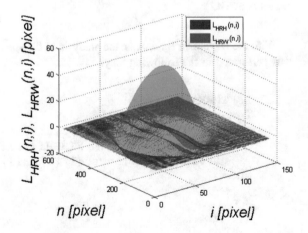

Fig. 4.14 Graph $L_{HRH}(n, i)$ in *black* and $L_{HRW}(n, i)$ in *blue*

```
[inte,ni]=max(max(LHR,[],2));
LHRT=LHR(ni,:);
Fs = 4330;
I = 140;
iFFT = 2^nextpow2(I);
f = Fs/2*linspace(0,1,iFFT/2+1);
LFFTHR = [fft(LHRT,iFFT)/I];
figure
bar(f,2*abs(LFFTHR(:,1:iFFT/2+1))','grouped');
ylabel('|L_{FFTHR}| [pix-
el]','FontSize',20,'FontAngle','Italic');
xlabel('f [Hz]','FontSize',20,'FontAngle','Italic');
axis([-10 400 0 38])
grid on
h6=ones(19);
LHRW=imresize(conv2(LHR,h6,'valid')/sum(h6(:)),size(LHR));
LHRH=LHR-LHRW;
figure;
hObj1=surfl(LHRH);
grid on; hold on
hObj2=surfl(LHRW);
xlabel('i [pixel]','FontSize',20,'FontAngle','Italic');
ylabel('n [pixel]','FontSize',20,'FontAngle','Italic');
zlabel('L_{HRH}(n,i), L_{HRW}(n,i) [pix-
el]','FontSize',20,'FontAngle','Italic');
shading interp
set(hObj1,'FaceColor',[0.2 0.2
0.2],'EdgeColor','none','FaceAlpha',0.3)
set(hObj2,'FaceColor',[0.3 0.3
0.9],'EdgeColor','none','FaceAlpha',0.3)
legend('L_{HRH}(n,i)', 'L_{HRW}(n,i)')
view(-50,42)
```

With the waveform $L_{HRH}(n, i)$, the analysis of the spectrum for each n-th column was performed in the following way:

```
LFFTHRH=[];
for n=1:size(LHRH,1)
    LFFTHRHi=fft(LHRH(n,:),iFFT)/I;
    LFFTHRHii=2*abs(LFFTHRHi(:,1:iFFT/2+1));
    LFFTHRH(n,1:length(LFFTHRHii))=LFFTHRHii;
end
```

```
f=f(1:30);
LFFTHRH=LFFTHRH(:,1:30);
[XX,YY]=meshgrid(f,1:size(LHR,1));
figure
surfl(XX,YY,LFFTHRH)
ylabel('n [pix-
el]','FontSize',20,'FontAngle','Italic');
zlabel('|L_{FFTHRH}| [pix-
el]','FontSize',20,'FontAngle','Italic');
xlabel('f [Hz]','FontSize',20,'FontAngle','Italic');
grid on
shading interp
colormap gray
view(-50,42)
```

The result is the waveform L_{FFTHRH} shown in Fig. 4.15

In the described case, due to the special shape of the waveform $L_{HR}(n, i)$, the provided method for measuring high frequencies does not produce the desired results. The reason are the areas of large signal derivatives occurring in the regions of two applanations. This problem is shown in Fig. 4.16 in black. In order to avoid this problem, the averaging filter should be replaced with the median filter, i.e.:

```
LHRW=imresize(conv2(LHR,h6,'valid')/sum(h6(:)),size(LH
R));
```

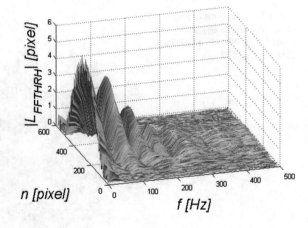

Fig. 4.15 Spectrum L_{FFTHRH} of the waveform $L_{HRH}(n, i)$ for $f \in (0.490)$ Hz using the function *conv2*

Fig. 4.16 Graph $L_{HRH}(n, i)$ with an artificial colour palette shown as a 2D image using the function *conv2*. The characteristic areas discussed in the text are marked in *black*

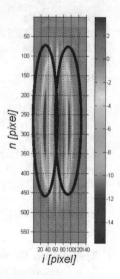

with:

```
LHRW=medfilt2(LHR,size(h6),'symmetric');
```

The proper spectrum L_{FFTHR} of the waveform $L_{HRH}(n, i)$ for $f \in (0.490)$ Hz and the graph $L_{HRH}(n, i)$ are shown in Figs. 4.17 and 4.18. The method of visualization of the spectrum L_{FFTHR} of the waveform $L_{HRH}(n, i)$ has also changed from the function *surfl* to *bar3*.

Fig. 4.17 Spectrum L_{FFTHRH} of the waveform $L_{HRH}(n, i)$ for $f \in (0.490)$ Hz using the function *medfilt2*

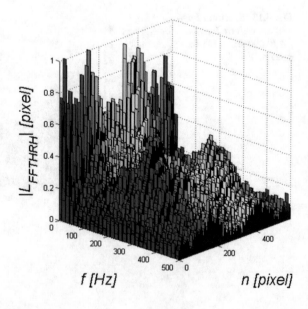

Fig. 4.18 Graph L_{HRH}
(n, i) with an artificial colour
palette shown as a 2D image
using the function *medfilt2*

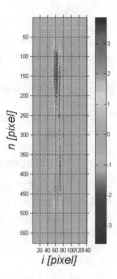

In the presented analyses and graphs, it is the numerical parameters that are important in medical diagnosis, which has been stressed many times before. In this case, the frequencies with the highest amplitude and their amplitude at two specific points of the graph $L_{HRH}(n, i)$ are vital. These points, n_L and n_R, are visible as local maxima on both sides of the mean amplitude (after i) shown in Fig. 4.19 and are obtained by means of fragments of the code which continue the previous notation:

Fig. 4.19 Graph $L_{HRHS}(n)$ as
a function of n and
automatically designated
points n_L and n_R

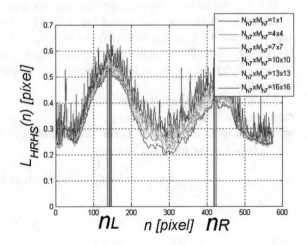

```
figure
colormap_=jet(16);
for Nh7=1:3:16
    Mh7=Nh7;
    LHRHS=mean(medfilt2(abs(LHRH),[Mh7
Nh7],'symmetric'),2);
    plot(LHRHS,'Color',colormap_(Nh7,:));
    grid on
    hold on
    [cc,nL]=max(LHRHS(1:round(length(LHRHS)/2)));

    [cc,nR]=max(LHRHS(round(length(LHRHS)/2)+1:end));
nR=nR+round(length(LHRHS)/2)+1;
    line([nL nR;nL nR], [0 0;max(LHRHS)
max(LHRHS)],'LineWidth',2,'Color',colormap_(Nh7,:));
end
xlabel('n
[pixel]','FontSize',20,'FontAngle','Italic');
ylabel('L_{HRHS}(n)
[pixel]','FontSize',20,'FontAngle','Italic');
hObj=findobj(gca,'Type','line');
legend(hObj(end:-
3:1),'N_{h7}xM_{h7}=1x1','N_{h7}xM_{h7}=4x4','N_{h7}xM
_{h7}=7x7','N_{h7}xM_{h7}=10x10','N_{h7}xM_{h7}=13x13'
,'N_{h7}xM_{h7}=16x16')
```

In the above code, in the next loop circuits, the size of the mask h_7 responsible for median filtering of the waveform L_{HRH} is changed in the range from $M_{h7} \times N_{h7} = 1 \times 1$ pixel (no filtration) to $M_{h7} \times N_{h7} = 16 \times 16$ pixels. This filtration is necessary due to the increased accuracy, repeatability of designating the points n_L and n_R. Finally, $M_{h7} \times N_{h7} = 16 \times 16$ pixels was adopted as the maximum size of the mask h_7.

Based on the designated position of the points n_L and n_R, time domain parameters are calculated:

$w(5)$ maximum difference between the minimum and maximum amplitude for each i at the point n_L, i.e.:

$$w(5) = \max_i L_{HRH}(n_L, i) - \min_i L_{HRH}(n_L, i) \qquad (4.19)$$

$w(6)$ maximum difference between the minimum and maximum amplitude for each i at the point n_R i.e.:

$$w(6) = \max_i L_{HRH}(n_R, i) - \min_i L_{HRH}(n_R, i) \qquad (4.20)$$

and frequency domain parameters:

$w(7)$ value of the maximum amplitude in the spectrum L_{FFTHRH} for $f \in (100,490)$ Hz at the point n_L,

$$w(7) = \max_f L_{FFTHRH}(n_L, f) \qquad (4.21)$$

$w(8)$ frequency value for the maximum amplitude in the spectrum L_{FFTHRH} for $f \in (100,490)$ Hz at the point n_L,

$$w(8) = \arg \max_f L_{FFTHRH}(n_L, f) \qquad (4.22)$$

$w(9)$ value of the maximum amplitude in the spectrum L_{FFTHRH} for $f \in (100,490)$ Hz at the point n_R,

$$w(9) = \max_f L_{FFTHRH}(n_R, f) \qquad (4.23)$$

w (10) frequency value for the maximum amplitude in the spectrum L_{FFTHRH} for $f \in (100,490)$ Hz at the point n_R,

$$w(10) = \arg \max_f L_{FFTHRH}(n_R, f) \qquad (4.24)$$

These parameters are calculated according to the following notation:

```
w5=max(LHRH(nL,:))-min(LHRH(nL,:));
w6=max(LHRH(nR,:))-min(LHRH(nR,:));
[w7,fi]=max(LFFTHRH(nL,6:end));
w8=f(fi+5);
[w9,fi]=max(LFFTHRH(nR,6:end));
w10=f(fi+5);
```

The adopted values "5" and "6" result directly from the value of the vector f which, in the analysed case, is:

```
f =
  Columns 1 through 4
   0   16.9   33.8   50.7
  Columns 5 through 8
   67.6   84.5   101.4   118.3
  Columns 9 through 12
   135.3   152.2   169.1   186.1 ...
```

The last three parameters $w(11)$, $w(12)$ and $w(13)$ concern directly the waveform L_{HRW} and are related to the value i for which the waveform L_{HRW} reaches its maximum:

$$w(11) = \arg \max_{n} \max_{n,i} L_{HRW}(n,i) \tag{4.25}$$

$$w(12) = \arg \max_{i} \max_{n,i} L_{HRW}(n,i) \tag{4.26}$$

$$w(13) = \max_{n,i} L_{HRW}(n,i) \tag{4.27}$$

The adequate source code is:

```
[cmm,maa]=max(LHRW,[],1);
[w13,w12]=max(cmm);
w11=maa(w12);
```

The obtained results, for example, graphs $L_{HOH}(i)$, $L_{HOW}(i)$, $L_{HRH}(i)$, $L_{HRW}(i)$ for $n = w(11)$, are shown in Fig. 4.20. These parameters are a further extension of the quantitative parameters defining the reaction of the eyeball and cornea to an air puff.

4.3.2   Determination of Applanation Points

One of the fundamental characteristics associated with the analysis of the corneal response to an air-puff are applanation points. Applanation is understood as temporary flattening of the cornea during the transition from a convex to concave state and vice versa. The moments in time at which applanation occurs can be measured

Fig. 4.20 Simplified graphs $L_{HOH}(i)$, $L_{HOW}(i)$, $L_{HRH}(i)$, $L_{HRW}(i)$ for $n = w(11)$

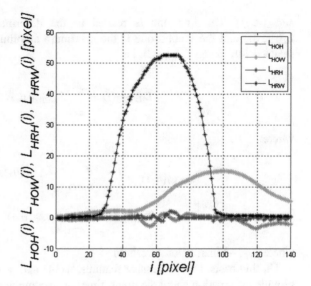

in accordance with the above definition. What is needed is the contour $L_{HRW}(n, i)$ where $i \in (1, I)$ for which the cornea gets flattened. Since the flattening of the cornea can occur at different angles relative to the image plane, it is necessary to apply the Radon transform. In the case of the image $L_{HRW}(n, i)$, the transform may be replaced by its modified version. This modification involves calculating the histogram for each row of the image $L_{HRW}(n, i)$. When flattening occurs, it will be visible as one top bar of the histogram, assuming that the flattening is perpendicular to the (horizontal) image plane. If this requirement is not met, the image $L_{HRW}(n, i)$ will have to undergo modifications before calculating histograms for subsequent i contours. This modification is based on the linear change in brightness of the successive image rows. It is performed by linear multiplication of the image $L_{HRW}(n, i)$ by the image $L_{HRWK}(n, i, \theta)$, i.e.:

$$L_{HRW2}(n, i, \theta) = L_{HRW}(n, i) \cdot L_{HRWK}(n, i, \theta) \tag{4.28}$$

where:

$$L_{HRWK}(n, i, \theta) = tg\theta \cdot (n - N/2) + \operatorname*{mean}_{n} L_{HRW}(n, i) \tag{4.29}$$

In practice, it is sufficient to analyse the histogram of the image $L_{HRWK}(n, i, \theta)$ in the range $\theta \in (-\pi/4, \pi/4)$. This method, however, requires tedious calculations of the histogram for each row of the image $L_{HRWK}(n, i, \theta)$ (which significantly overloads CPU). It is much easier in this case to use two features of the image

$L_{HRW}(n, i)$. The first one is related to the deformation length measured as $L_{HRWBS}(i)$ and the second one is the maximum amplitude of deformation for the selected i-th image $L_{HRWM}(i)$. i.e.:

$$L_{HRWBS}(i) = \sum_{n=1}^{N} L_{HRWB}(n, i) \qquad (4.30)$$

where:

$$L_{HRWB}(n, i) = \begin{cases} 1 & if \quad L_{HRW}(n, i) > p_{r13} \\ 0 & other \end{cases} \qquad (4.31)$$

$$L_{HRWM}(i) = \max_{n} L_{HRW}(n, i) \qquad (4.32)$$

where p_{r13}—binarization threshold.

On this basis, two successive features, $w(14)$ and $w(15)$, are determined which provide information about the point (time) of two applanations (before and after the moment when the maximum deformation occurred—$w(12)$):

$$w(14) = arg \max_{i\epsilon(1, w(12))} \left(\frac{L_{HRWBS}(i)}{L_{HRWM}(i)} \right) \qquad (4.33)$$

$$w(15) = arg \max_{i\epsilon(w(12)+1, I)} \left(\frac{L_{HRWBS}(i)}{L_{HRWM}(i)} \right) \qquad (4.34)$$

The idea of this measurement is shown in Fig. 4.21.

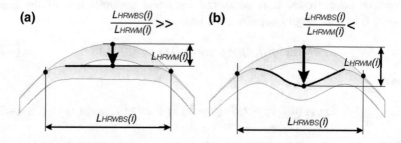

Fig. 4.21 Idea of applanation point measurement

The corresponding source code is shown below:

```
colormap_=jet(16);
figure
for pr13=1:10
    LHRWBS=sum(LHRW>pr13);
    LHRWM=max(LHRW);
    plot(LHRWBS./LHRWM,'Color',colormap_(pr13,:))
    hold on
    grid on

[~,w14]=max(LHRWBS(1:round(length(LHRWBS)/2))./LHRWM(1
:round(length(LHRWM)/2)));

[~,w15]=max(LHRWBS(round(length(LHRWBS)/2)+1:end)./LHR
WM(round(length(LHRWM)/2)+1:end));
    w15=w15+round(length(LHRWM)/2);
    line([w14 w15;w14 w15], [0 0;max(LHRWBS./LHRWM)
max(LHRWBS./LHRWM)],'LineWidth',2,'Color',colormap_(pr
13,:));
end
xlabel('i [pix-
el]','FontSize',20,'FontAngle','Italic');
ylabel('L_{HRWBS}(i)/L_{HRWM}(i)
[/]','FontSize',20,'FontAngle','Italic');
hObj=findobj(gca,'Type','line');
legend(hObj(end:-
3:1),'p_{r13}=1','p_{r13}=2','p_{r13}=3','p_{r13}=4','
p_{r13}=5','p_{r13}=6','p_{r13}=7','p_{r13}=8','p_{r13
}=9','p_{r13}=10')
```

The impact of the binarization threshold p_{r13} on the results was analysed—values of the features $w(14)$ and $w(15)$. The obtained results are shown on the graph in Figs. 4.22 and 4.23.

The graph (Fig. 4.22) shows that the maximum amplitude is obtained for the binarization threshold $p_{r13} = 1$. Changing the threshold value to $p_{r13} = 2$ or $p_{r13} = 3$ alters the results obtained—the values of $w(14)$ and $w(15)$ are then in the range ± 1 (Fig. 4.23). Therefore, $p_{r13} = 1$ was adopted for further considerations. The duration

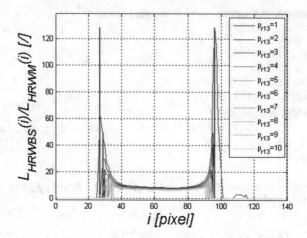

Fig. 4.22 Graph of changes in $L_{HRWBS}(i)/L_{HRWM}(i)$ for successive i images (pixels) and different threshold values, $p_{r13} \in (1,10)$

p_{r13}	1	2	3	4	5	6	7
$w(14)$	27	29	30	32	32	34	34
$w(15)$	96	95	94	94	94	93	93

Fig. 4.23 Summary of changes in the values of $w(14)$ and $w(15)$ for the threshold $p_{r13} \in (1, 7)$

of the points (moments) of applanation is also vital (for the features $w(14)$ and $w(15)$) (see Fig. 4.21). As a result, additional features $w(16)$ and $w(17)$ were determined, defined in the source code as:

```
w16=LHRWBS(w14);
w17=LHRWBS(w15);
```

The features $w(16)$ and $w(17)$ further complement the existing features.

4.3.3   3D Reconstruction

The measurements performed with the use of the Corvis tonometer concern only one section of the cornea in the horizontal axis. Due to the nature of tonometer operation, there is no information about the location and changes in the cornea in other places. However, having information about the properties of the cornea,

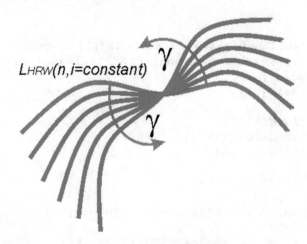

Fig. 4.24 Idea of 3D reconstruction performed on the basis of the selected corneal. contour $L_{HRH}(n, i)$ or $L_{HRW}(n, i)$ for a constant n. The contour of known location is shown in *red*. The reconstructed contour position resulting from rotation of the corneal contour ($L_{HRH}(n, i)$ or $L_{HRW}(n, i)$) is marked in *green*

mainly its allowable curvature and position changes, it is possible to try to perform its 3D reconstruction. The use of reconstruction in this case cannot be in any way related to metrology. It is only an attempt to better understand the phenomena occurring in response to an air-puff. The basis for further analyses will be the images $L_{HRH}(n, i)$ and $L_{HRW}(n, i)$ and, to be more specific, the selected waveforms for the chosen i (Fig. 4.14). The ideas of 3D reconstruction are shown in Fig. 4.24.

The idea of 3D reconstruction (Fig. 4.24) involves rotation of the corneal contour $L_{HRH}(n, i)$ or $L_{HRW}(n, i)$ around the main axis of the cornea for a constant n (the contour marked in red—Fig. 4.24). The range of angular values γ (Fig. 4.24) is closely dependent on the reconstruction accuracy. In the analysed cases, it was adopted that $\gamma \in (0, 2\pi)$. Figure 4.24 shows in green the reconstructed contour position resulting from rotation of the corneal contour ($L_{HRH}(n, i)$ or $L_{HRW}(n, i)$) by an angle $\gamma \in \{10, 20, 30, 40\}$ degrees. The missing information related to rotation was calculated using linear interpolation—*linspace* function. Assuming further that the resulting image is $L_{HRH3D}(n, v, i)$, the analysis is carried out for a particular i-th image $L_{HRH}(n, i)$. Below there is a sample source code which enables to obtain 3D reconstruction for $i = 67$:

```
i=67;
n=(1:length(LHRH(:,i)))'; nm=mean(n); n=n-nm;
z=LHRH(:,i); z=conv2(z,ones([19 1]),'same')/19;
zf=flipud(z);
v=zeros(size(z));
de=[];
for i=1:length(zf)
    pd=linspace(z(i),zf(i),360);
    de(1:360,i)=pd;
end
nn=[]; vv=[]; LHRH3D=[];
for ga=1:1:360
    [THETA,PHI,R]=cart2sph(n,v,de(ga,:)');
    THETA=THETA+ga/360*pi;
    [n2,v2,z2] = sph2cart(THETA,PHI,R);
    nn(1:length(n),ga)=n2+nm;
    vv(1:length(v),ga)=v2+nm;
    LHRH3D(1:length(z),ga)=z2;
end
figure; surf(nn,vv,LHRH3D,'FaceColor','interp',...
 'EdgeColor','none',...
 'FaceLighting','phong')
axis tight
view(-6,30)
camlight left
camlight right
set(gca,'ZDir','reverse')
hold on
plot3(n+nm,v+nm,z,'-r*')
xlabel('n [pixel]','FontSize',20,'FontAngle','italic')
ylabel('v [pixel]','FontSize',20,'FontAngle','italic')
zlabel('L_{HRW3D}(n,v,i) [pix-
el]','FontSize',20,'FontAngle','italic')
```

The results obtained are shown in Fig. 4.25. The original contour for $L_{HRH}(n, i)$ for $i = 67$ is marked in red. The results obtained for other values are shown in Fig. 4.26. 3D reconstruction for the selected contour of the image $L_{HRH}(n, i)$ (for example $i = 67$) can be performed in the same way, which is presented in Fig. 4.27.

At this point I encourage readers to carry out reconstruction for different, selected, subsequent values i. It would be also interesting to investigate the effect of the size of mask h_6 (the default size is $M_{h6} \times N_{h6} = 19 \times 19$ pixels) on the results obtained.

Fig. 4.25 Result of 3D reconstruction (image $L_{HRH3D}(n, v, i)$) performed on the basis of information for the selected corneal contour ($L_{HRH}(n, i)$) for $i = 67$

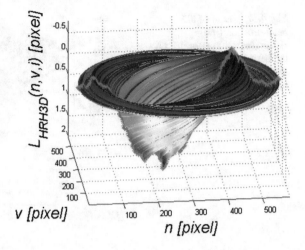

Fig. 4.26 Result of 3D reconstruction (image $L_{HRH3D}(n,v,i)$) performed on the basis of information for the selected corneal contour ($L_{HRH}(n, i)$) for: **a** $i = 65$; **b** $i = 66$; **c** $i = 67$; **d** $i = 68$

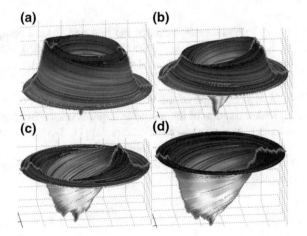

4.3.4 Response Analysis

Analysis of the corneal response to an air-puff is a relatively difficult issue. On the one hand, it is necessary to remove the eyeball reaction (as shown in the previous chapters). On the other hand, it is necessary to designate the shape of the force and type of the object which is the cornea. As proven in works [1, 3–5] the force (an air-puff) acting directly on the cornea in its main axis has the following form:

$$F_{ap}(i) = \underbrace{F_1 \cdot exp\left[-\frac{(i-i_1)^2}{2 \cdot \sigma_1^2}\right]}_{I} + \underbrace{F_2 \cdot exp\left[-\frac{(i-i_2)^2}{2 \cdot \sigma_2^2}\right]}_{II} \qquad (4.35)$$

Fig. 4.27 Result of 3D reconstruction (image $L_{HRW3D}(n, v, i)$) performed on the basis of information for the selected corneal contour ($L_{HRW}(n, i)$) for $i = 67$

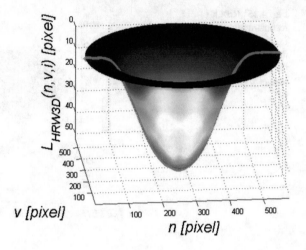

where:

F_1, F_2 pressure amplitude of the first and second component,
i_1, i_2 the mean value of the time shift of the first and second component,
σ_1, σ_2 standard deviation of the first and second component

A typical shape of the pressure applied to the cornea is shown in Fig. 4.28.

Determination of the response requires presenting a typical cornea in the form of a model. According to the literature data [1, 3–5], the cornea can be represented as a second-order inertia object—Fig. 4.29.

The equation of the dynamics of the system shown in Fig. 4.29 can be written as follows:

$$c_m \cdot \frac{d^2 L_{HRW}(i)}{di^2} + b \cdot \frac{d L_{HRW}(i)}{di} + k \cdot L_{HRW}(i) = A \cdot F_{ap}(i) \qquad (4.36)$$

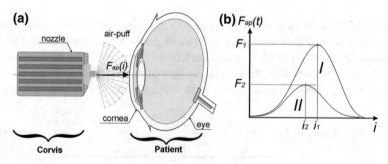

Fig. 4.28 Schematic diagram of the impact of an air-puff on the cornea (**a**) and a typical shape of the pressure applied to the cornea during the measurement (**b**)

Fig. 4.29 Schematic diagram of force $F_{ap}(i)$ and intraocular pressure (*IOP*) (**a**) and a dynamic model (**b**)

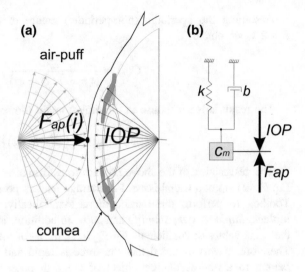

where:

c_m corneal mass,
b shock absorber constant,
k spring resilience constant,
A amplification factor

When simplified, the above formula takes the following form:

$$\frac{d^2 L_{HRW}(i)}{di^2} + \frac{b}{c_m} \cdot \frac{dL_{HRW}(i)}{di} + \frac{k}{c_m} \cdot L_{HRW}(i) = \frac{A}{c_m} \cdot F_{ap}(i) \qquad (4.37)$$

For zero initial points the equation can be written as operators:

$$s^2 \cdot L_{HRW}(s) + \frac{b}{c_m} \cdot s \cdot L_{HRW}(s) + \frac{k}{c_m} \cdot L_{HRW}(s) = \frac{A}{c_m} \cdot F_{ap}(s) \qquad (4.38)$$

Hence the transfer function:

$$G(s) = \frac{L_{HRW}(s)}{F_{ap}(s)} = \frac{\frac{A}{c_m}}{s^2 + \frac{b}{c_m} \cdot s + \frac{k}{c_m}} \qquad (4.39)$$

Zero points are calculated based on the equation:

$$s_{1,2} = -\frac{b}{2c_m} \pm \sqrt{\left(\frac{b}{2c_m}\right)^2 - \frac{k}{c_m}} \qquad (4.40)$$

Assuming the aperiodic (non-periodic) nature of the impulse response, i.e. $b > 2\,k$, we obtain:

$$G(s) = \frac{\frac{A}{c_m}}{(s - s_1) \cdot (s - s_2)} \qquad (4.41)$$

The result is the response in the time domain (domain i) $L_{HRW}(i)$, i.e.:

$$L_{HRW}(i) = \mathcal{L}^{-1}\{G(s)F_{ap}(s)\} \qquad (4.42)$$

The designation of the above Laplace transform after substituting values into the Eq. (4.42) is not a trivial issue. I encourage readers possessing the Symbolic Math Toolbox to perform these calculations symbolically. The needed features are: *laplace, ilaplace, sym, simplify* and *subs*. In addition, in the above considerations, the exact values of coefficients F_1, F_2, i_1, i_2, σ_1, σ_2 of the Eq. (4.35) are not known. Therefore, it was assumed that the force is rapid and the recognized parameters belong to a non-oscillating object of the q-th order containing the delay. The assumptions significantly simplify the model and form of the force but allow for the use of a simple method to estimate the basic parameters of the response $L_{HRW}(i)$.

The use of the Strejc's method for the response $L_{HRW}(i)$ resulted in:

setting a tangent at the inflection point T_A.

- determination of the first inflection point T_A of the waveform $L_{HRW}(i)$,
- determination of the tangent at the inflection point T_A,
- determination of the model row based on the calculated ratio $T_m/(T_z - T_m)$ (see Fig. 4.30) and reading the model row from the table [2],
- recording the final form of the model.

This method (Strejc's method) requires the use of a table for determining the order of the model. An interesting idea is to use approximation of the model of the

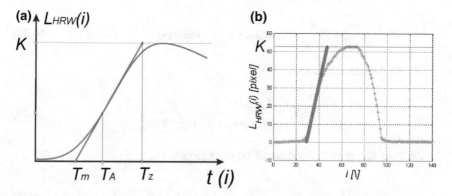

Fig. 4.30 Method for calculating the parameters of an inertia object of the q-th order using the Strejc's approach and simplifying the inertia object of the q-th order to the object of the first order with the transport delay (**a**) the corresponding result of the calculations using the proposed algorithm (**b**)

q-th order with the first-order model with the transport delay $T_z - T_m$. Therefore, it is possible to propose the transfer function (4.39) modified to the form created on the basis of the experiment results, i.e.:

$$G(s) \cong \frac{K}{T_z \cdot s + 1} \cdot e^{-s(T_z - T_m)} \tag{4.43}$$

In the analysed case, the transfer function takes the following form:

$$G(s) \cong \frac{52.66}{29.01 \cdot s + 1} \cdot e^{-s17.77} \tag{4.44}$$

where:

K 52.66 pixels,
T_z 29.01 of the image, i.e. 29.01 × 231 μs,
$T_z - T_m$ 17.77 of the image, i.e. 17.77 × 231 μs

In this model, the obtained time constants are intuitive and easy to interpret:

- the gain value K is the maximum calculated from $L_{HRW}(i)$,
- the time constant $T_z - T_m$ results directly from the rate of corneal response to the force,
- the time constant T_z is the transport delay calculated from the beginning of data registration (and not from the beginning of force application as it should be) which gives a specific and reproducible feature of the dynamics of corneal response to force.

The corresponding fragment of the source code is shown below:

```
y2=LHRW(282,:);
[C,I]=max(diff(y2));
k=(mean(diff(y2(I-1:I+1))))/(mean(diff(x2(I-1:I+1))));
b=y2(I)-k*x2(I);
xz=min(x2):0.01:max(x2);
yz=k*xz+b;
xy=[xz(:), yz(:)];
xy(xy(:,2)<0,:)=[];
xy(xy(:,2)>max(y2),:)=[];
Tm=xy(1,1);
Tz=xy(end,1);
plot(xy(:,1),xy(:,2),'-r*')
grid on
line([1 140],[max(y2) max(y2)]);
xlabel('i [\]','FontSize',20,'FontAngle','italic')
ylabel('L_{HRW}(i) [pix-
el]','FontSize',20,'FontAngle','italic')
```

On this basis, the next two features $w(18)$ and $w(19)$ are calculated, which are defined as time constants T_m and $T_z - T_m$.

4.3.5   Symmetry Analysis

Corneal response symmetry analysis concerns the quantitative analysis of differences in response between the left and right part of the cornea. The analysis is carried out for each i-th image. The idea of measurement is shown in Fig. 4.31.

According to the idea of measurement shown in Fig. 4.31, the use of the above measured value of the feature $w(11)$ results in the calculation of the difference:

$$L_{DHRW}(n_D, i) = L_{HRW}(n_D, i) - L_{HRW}(N - n_D, i) \tag{4.45}$$

where: $n_D \in (1, w(11))$.

The differences for the waveform $L_{HR}(n, i)$ were calculated providing $L_{DHR}(n_D, i)$. The waveforms $L_{DHR}(n_D, i)$ and $L_{DHRW}(n_D, i)$ are shown in Fig. 4.32.

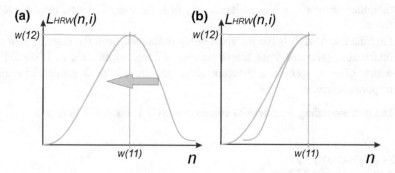

Fig. 4.31 Graph $L_{HRW}(i)$ as a function of i (**a**) and demonstrative graph of symmetry analysis (**b**)

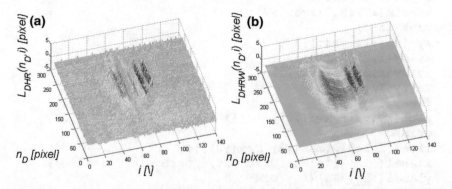

Fig. 4.32 Graph $L_{DHR}(n_D, i)$ (**a**) and $L_{DHRW}(n_D, i)$ (**b**)

On this basis, the next feature $w(20)$ is measured:

$$w(20) = \max_{n_D,i} L_{DHRW}(n_D, i) - \min_{n_D,i} L_{DHRW}(n_D, i) \tag{4.46}$$

In the above calculations it is quite important to accurately calculate the feature $w(11)$. Figure 4.33 below shows the effect of the accuracy of calculating the feature $w(11)$ on the value of $w(20)$.

The adequate fragment of the source code:

```
[cmm,maa]=max(LHRW,[],1);
[w13,w12]=max(cmm);
w11=maa(w12);
figure;
mesh(LHR(1:w11,:)-LHR(2*(w11-1):-1:(w11-1),:))
xlabel('i [\]','FontSize',20,'FontAngle','italic')
ylabel('n_D [pixel]','FontSize',20,'FontAngle','italic')
zlabel('L_{DHR}(n_D,i) [pix-
el]','FontSize',20,'FontAngle','italic')
view(-16,74)
figure;
mesh(LHRW(1:w11,:)-LHRW(2*(w11-1):-1:(w11-1),:))
xlabel('i [\]','FontSize',20,'FontAngle','italic')
ylabel('n_D [pixel]','FontSize',20,'FontAngle','italic')
zlabel('L_{DHRW}(n_D,i) [pix-
el]','FontSize',20,'FontAngle','italic')
view(-16,74)
pam=[];pam2=[];
for id=(w11-38):(w11+10)
    LDHRW=LHRW(1:id,:)-LHRW(2*(id-1):-1:(id-1),:);
    LDHR=LHR(1:id,:)-LHR(2*(id-1):-1:(id-1),:);
    pam=[pam;[id, max(LDHRW(:))-min(LDHRW(:)) ]];
    pam2=[pam2;[id, max(LDHR(:))-min(LDHR(:)) ]];
end
figure; plot(pam(:,1),pam(:,2),'-b*'); hold on; grid on
plot(pam2(:,1),pam2(:,2),'-g*');
xlabel('w(11) [pixel]','FontSize',20,'FontAngle','italic')
ylabel('w(20) [pixel]','FontSize',20,'FontAngle','italic')
```

The graph in Fig. 4.33 shows high sensitivity of the feature $w(20)$ to changes in w (11). It results directly from the idea of measurement shown in Fig. 4.31. For the value of $w(11)$ oscillating around the 275-th pixel (Fig. 4.33), the constant component shown in Fig. 4.32 does not affect the result. Significantly smaller or greater values of $w(11)$ (above the 275-th pixel—Fig. 4.33) result in a significant effect of the constant component. It affects the result linearly by falsifying it. However, this fact does not affect in any way the obtained results since the value of $w(11)$ is calculated automatically (its sourcing methodology was discussed several chapters above).

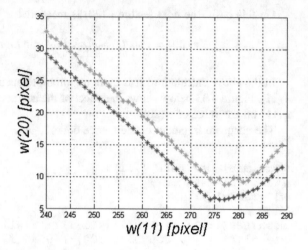

Fig. 4.33 Graph of changes in the value of $w(20)$ as a function of changes in the value of $w(11)$. *Green*—graph $L_{DHR}(n_D, i)$ and *blue*—graph $L_{DHRW}(n_D, i)$

4.4   Summary of Image Processing

The individual blocks of image processing discussed in the previous subchapters are shown in Fig. 4.34.

The individual blocks in Fig. 4.34 were not implemented in Matlab. Fragments or the full source code enabling to obtain individual results, in particular the values of features from $w(1)$ to $w(20)$, are shown in the following subchapters. However, in practice, the use of this code is cumbersome because of the lack of a graphical user interface (GUI). Therefore, as in the case of image pre-processing, the GUI implementation shown below was proposed.

The GUI of the full application is directly related to image pre-processing described above. Therefore, the description presented below is a supplement and extension of the GUI outlined in Sect. 2.5. As some of the functions are duplicated (*CorvisGUI.m* and *CorvisFunction*) in relation to Sect. 2.5, they were separated by saving them in two separate folders (*zip* containers) attached to this monograph:

- folder *pre_processing* containing functions related only to image pre-processing,
- folder *processing* containing functions related to full image processing.

The full GUI with functions intended for analysis and processing was implemented in six m-files (folder *processing*):

CorvisGUI.m	responsible for placement of buttons, images, and other menu items,
CorvisFunction.m	responsible for the type and form of response to pressing a button or another action of the user,
CorvisCalcPre.m	image pre-processing function,
CorvisCalcMain.m	function intended for main image processing,

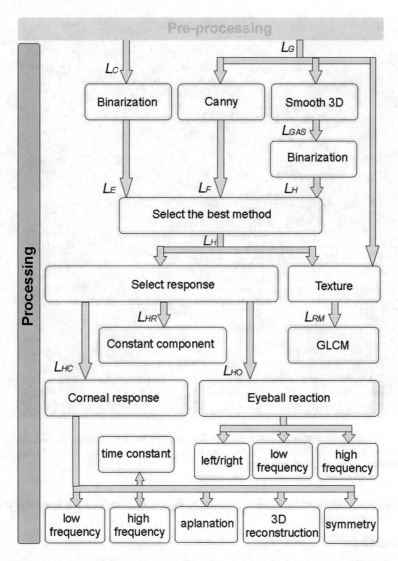

Fig. 4.34 Block diagram of individual stages of image processing. Details of image pre-processing were omitted and replaced with a single block (they were discussed in detail in Chap. 2)

Corvis_Method.m   function designed to select the desired main processing method (discussed in Chap. 3 Main image processing)
CorvisExcel_write.m function designed to write selected results to an Excel file

The main window of the application developed using the six m-files is shown in Fig. 4.35.

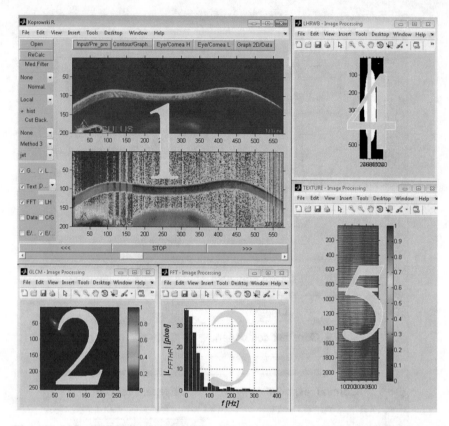

Fig. 4.35 Main application window (GUI)—full program version (1) together with additional windows: (2) GLCM window; (3) FFT window; (4) window of the binary image L_{HRW}; (5) window containing the corneal texture

The main application window shown in Fig. 4.35 consists of a few new characteristic elements:

- checkbox:

    - *GLCM*—showing or hiding window 2—Fig. 4.35,
    - *LHRWB*—showing or hiding window 4—Fig. 4.35,
    - *Texture*—showing or hiding window 5—Fig. 4.35,
    - *FFT*—showing or hiding window 3—Fig. 4.35
    - *LH*—recording the image L_H in the form of tabular data in the Excel file *FileName_LH.xls*,

- *Data*—recordning the features from $w(1)$ to $w(20)$ in the form of tabular data in the Excel file *FileName_w.xls*,
- *E/CL*—recording images L_{HOW} and L_{HRW} in the Excel files *FileName_LHOW.xls* and *FileName_LHRW.xls*;
- *E/CH*—recodring images L_{HOH} and L_{HRH} in the Excel files *FileName_LHOH.xls* and *FileName_LHRH.xls*,
- *C/G*—recording waveforms L_{HOW}, L_{HRW}, L_{HOH} and L_{HRH} but only for $w(11)$ in the form of tabular data in the Excel file *FileName_LH_O_R_H_W.xls*,

- pop-up menus:

  - changing the threshold p_{r9} in the range from 4 to 20 every 1;
  - choosing the processing method: *Method1, Method2* or *Method 3*,
  - choosing the colour palette—*jet, hot, hsv, prism, flag* or *gray*,

- push buttons:

  - *Input/Pre_pro*—choosing the window with the input image and the image resulting from image pre-processing,
  - *Contour/Graph3D*—choosing the window with the image of the corneal contour for the analysed 2D image (specific *i*) and the 3D graph of the outer corneal contour,
  - *Eye/Cornea H*—choosing the window with the 3D graph of the corneal contour response and eyeball reaction for high frequencies (L_{HOH} and L_{HRH}),
  - *Eye/Cornea L*—choosing the window with the 3D graph of the corneal contour response and eyeball reaction for low frequencies (L_{HOW} and L_{HRW}),
  - *Graph 2D/Data*—choosing the 2D graph of the waveforms L_{HOW}, L_{HRW}, L_{HOH} and L_{HRH} but only for $w(11)$ and numerical data for the selected i-th image (bottom left) and for the whole sequence (bottom right)

The other menu items were shown and described in detail in the chapter on image pre-processing. The new menu items and additional functionality are an extension of the elements from image pre-processing (Fig. 2.10). Consequently, in the variable *hObj* there are handles of individual GUI elements. The work with the program starts by clicking the button *Open*. Selection of one of the **.jpg* images from a sequence or an **.avi* file is followed by its processing and analysis. At that time, the noise in images 2, 3, 4, 5 (Fig. 4.35) is shown. After the analysis, which lasts a few seconds depending on the processor speed, it is possible to browse the created 2D and 3D graphs by pressing the buttons at the top of the menu: *Input/Pre_pro, Contour/Graph3D, Eye/Cornea H Eye/Cornea L* or *Graph 2D/ Data*. For each of the displayed 2D or 3D images, a line (blue or yellow) indicating

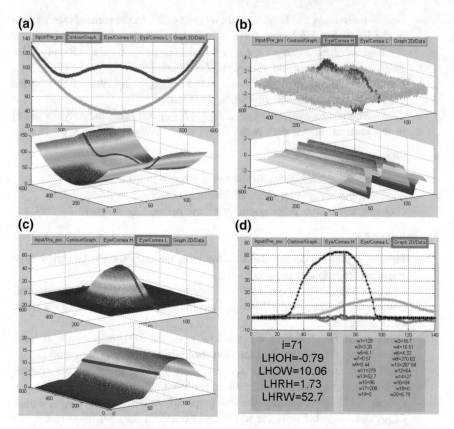

Fig. 4.36 Four sets of graphs and data dependent on pressing the buttons: **a** *Contour/Graph3D*; **b** *Eye/Cornea H*; **c** *Eye/Cornea L*; **d** *Graph 2D/Data*

the current viewed image was additionally shown. The four new windows are shown in Fig. 4.36.

If the checkbox fields are selected, the images L_H, L_{HOW}, L_{HRW}, L_{HOH} and L_{HRH} as well as the values of features w are automatically saved to Excel files. These files are named the same as the input files from the Corvis tonometer and the end of their names is associated with the content of the saved file (*_w.xls, *._LHRW.xls, *._LHRW.xls, *._LHRW.xls, *._LHRW.xls or *_LH.xls). The structure of Excel files is consistent with successive pixel values for individual rows and columns of the matrix, and in the case of recording the features w, in order of their occurrence. The application was written using all parts of the algorithm discussed in previous chapters. The full uniformity concerning the names of variables present in the source code of the described application was retained in accordance with the names of variables adopted in this monograph. The structure of all m-files will not be discussed here in detail because of its large volume, except for two files: *CorvisExcel_write* and *CorvisCalcMain*. The *CorvisExcel_write* file is the smallest of these files and enables to save data to Excel files using the following source code:

```
function CorvisExcel_write
global hObj PathName FileName LEFH LHRH LHRW LHOH LHOW w

if get(hObj(68),'Value') %LH'
        xlswrite([PathName,FileName,'_LH.xls'],LEFH);
end
if get(hObj(65),'Value') %C/G'
    CG=[];
    CG=[CG;LHRH(w(11),:)];
    CG=[CG;LHOH(w(11),:)];
    CG=[CG;LHRW(w(11),:)];
    CG=[CG;LHOW(w(11),:)];
        xlswrite([PathName,FileName,'_LH_O_R_H_W.xls'],CG);
end
if get(hObj(67),'Value') %E/CH
        xlswrite([PathName,FileName,'_LHRH.xls'],LHRH);
        xlswrite([PathName,FileName,'_LHOH.xls'],LHOH);
end
if get(hObj(66),'Value') % E/CL
        xlswrite([PathName,FileName,'_LHRW.xls'],LHRW);
        xlswrite([PathName,FileName,'_LHOW.xls'],LHOW);
end
if get(hObj(64),'Value') % Data
        xlswrite([PathName,FileName,'_w.xls'],w);
end
```

As is apparent from the given source code, depending on the value indicated by the user and thus the values read using the handles from *hObj(64)* to *hObj(68)*, there follows an appropriate response—record to the **.xls file*. These handles (from *hObj (64)* to *hObj(68)*) are associated with checkbox elements created in the *CorvisGUI. m* file, i.e.:

```
...
hObj(64)=uicontrol('Style', 'check-
box','units','normalized','FontUnits','normalized',
'String','Data','Value',1,'Position', [0.001 0.16 0.07
0.07],'BackgroundColor',col,'Callback', 'CorvisFunc-
tion(19)','Parent',hObj(1));
hObj(65)=uicontrol('Style', 'check-
box','units','normalized','FontUnits','normalized',
'String','C/G','Value',1,'Position', [0.071 0.16 0.07
0.07],'BackgroundColor',col,'Callback', 'CorvisFunc-
tion(19)','Parent',hObj(1));
hObj(66)=uicontrol('Style', 'check-
box','units','normalized','FontUnits','normalized',
'String','E/CL','Value',1,'Position', [0.001 0.09 0.07
0.07],'BackgroundColor',col,'Callback', 'CorvisFunc-
tion(19)','Parent',hObj(1));
hObj(67)=uicontrol('Style', 'check-
box','units','normalized','FontUnits','normalized',
'String','E/CH','Value',1,'Position', [0.071 0.09 0.07
0.07],'BackgroundColor',col,'Callback', 'CorvisFunc-
tion(19)','Parent',hObj(1));
hObj(68)=uicontrol('Style', 'check-
box','units','normalized','FontUnits','normalized',
'String','LH','Value',1,'Position', [0.071 0.23 0.07
0.07],'BackgroundColor',col,'Callback', 'CorvisFunc-
tion(19)','Parent',hObj(1));
...
```

As is apparent from the above source code fragment of the *CorvisGUI.m* file, individual *checkbox* elements differ mainly in terms of position ('Position' [....]). It should be noted that it is the relative position expressed as a percentage. The first two values represent the position of the lower left corner of the menu item, while the next two are the values of its size in the x and y axes. An example of writing the data to *_LH_O_R_H_W.xls* with the use of the *CorvisExcel_write* function is shown in Fig. 4.37.

The second discussed function is *CorvisCalcMain*. It enables to perform the main image processing. It consists of a few elements. The first one concerns texture analysis, the second—FFT calculation, and the third—calculation of symmetry and determination of the other values of features w. The input arguments for the *CorvisCalcMain* function are virtually all matrices obtained from image pre-processing (from the CorvisCalcPre function). The CorvisCalcMain function analyzes all the results obtained from the application. In particular, these are L_{HC}, L_{HHC}, L_{HO}, L_{HR}, L_{HRH}, L_{HRW}, L_{HOH}, L_{HOW}, L_{GK}, L_{FFTHRH}, L_{FFTHR}, L_{GLCM}, L_{HRWB}, w. When the user selected method 3 of corneal contour analysis, it was necessary to introduce a global variable L_{GA} (see Sect. 3.4). This is due to the need to supplement

Fig. 4.37 Fragment of writing the data of L_{HOW}, L_{HRW}, L_{HOH} and L_{HRH} for $w(11)$ to the Excel file (*_LH_O_R_H_W.xls)

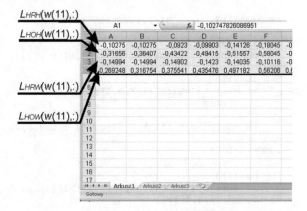

the L_{GA} matrix in each iteration (each call for subsequent i) of the *CorvisCalcMain* function. The full source code of the *CorvisCalcMain* function is shown below:

```
function
[LHC,LHHC,LHO,LHR,LHRH,LHRW,LHOH,LHOW,LGK,f,LFFTHRH,LFFTHR,
iFFT,LGLCM,LHRWB,w]=CorvisCalcMain(LMED,LRM,LQ,LC,ContMe,LH
)
global LGA pr
w=zeros(1,20);
%%%%%%%%%%%%%%%%%%%%%%%%%%%%%%%%%%%%%%%% texture
pr10=0.001;   LGK=[];
pr9=pr(9);
for ii=1:size(LH,2)
    LGK_=[];
    for n=1:size(LH,1)
        Lp=round(LH(n,ii)); Lp(Lp<1)=1;
        Lk=round(LH(n,ii)+pr9-1);
Lk(Lk>size(LH,2))=size(LH,2);
        LGK_(1:(Lk-Lp+1),n)=LGA(n,ii,Lp:Lk);
    end
    LGK=[LGK;LGK_];
end
LGKS=mean(LGK',1);
LGKSM=medfilt2(LGKS,[1 19],'symmetric');
LBIN3=((LGKS<(LGKSM+pr10))&(LGKS>(LGKSM-pr10)))';
LGB=LGK;
LGB(LBIN3==0,:)=[];
if (min(size(LGB))>1) && (~isempty(LGB))
    saa=10; saa(saa>size(LGB,1))=size(LGB,1)-1;
    LGLCM = graycomatrix(uint8(round(LGB*255)),'Offset',[-
saa 0],'NumLevels',256);
    LBIN4=LGLCM>1;
    LBIN5=imrotate(LBIN4,45,'nearest');
    w(1)=sum(sum(LBIN5,2)>0);
else
    w(1)=0;
end
%%%%%%%%%%%%%%%%%%%%%%%%%%%%%%%%%%%%%%%%
```

```matlab
LH=medfilt2(LH,[3 3],'symmetric');
pam=[];
for is=1:size(LH,2)
    pam=[pam;[is, max(std(LH(:,1:is),0,2))]];
end
for is=1:10
    if max(std(LH(:,1:is),0,2))>1
        break
    end
    LHC=mean(LH(:,1:is),2)*ones([1 size(LH,2)]);
end
LHHC=LH-LHC;

for ns=1:10
    if (max(std(LHHC(1:ns,:),0,1))>1)|(max(std(LHHC((end-
ns-1):end,:),0,1))>1)
        if ns>1
            break
        end
    end
    LP=mean(LHHC(1:ns,:),1);

    LK=mean(LHHC((end-ns-1):end,:),1);
    LHO=[];
    for i=1:length(LP)
LHO(1:size(LHHC,1),i)=linspace(LP(i),LK(i),size(LHHC,1));
    end
end
LHR=LHHC-LHO;
 [inte,ni]=max(max(LHR,[],2));
 LHRT=LHR(ni,:);
 Fs = 4330;
 I = 140;
 iFFT = 2^nextpow2(I);
 f = Fs/2*linspace(0,1,iFFT/2+1);
 LFFTHR = [fft(LHRT,iFFT)/I];
%%%%%%%%%%%%%%%%%%%%%%%%%%%%%% FILTER %%%%%%%%%%%%%%%%%%%%%%
h6=ones(19);
LHRW=medfilt2(LHR,size(h6),'symmetric');
LHRH=LHR-LHRW;
    pr13=1;
    LHRWBS=sum(LHRW>pr13);
    LHRWB=LHRW>pr13;
    LHRWM=max(LHRW);
[~,w14]=max(LHRWBS(1:round(length(LHRWBS)/2))./LHRWM(1:roun
d(length(LHRWM)/2)));
[~,w15]=max(LHRWBS(round(length(LHRWBS)/2)+1:end)./LHRWM(ro
und(length(LHRWM)/2)+1:end));
```

```
      w15=w15+round(length(LHRWM)/2);
      w(14)=w14;
      w(15)=w15;
      w(16)=LHRWBS(w14);
      w(17)=LHRWBS(w15);
LFFTHRH=[];
for n=1:size(LHRH,1)
        LFFTHRHi=fft(LHRH(n,:),iFFT)/I;
        LFFTHRHii=2*abs(LFFTHRHi(:,1:iFFT/2+1));
        LFFTHRH(n,1:length(LFFTHRHii))=LFFTHRHii;
end
f=f(1:30);
LFFTHRH=LFFTHRH(:,1:30);
Nh7=3;
Mh7=Nh7;
LHRHS=mean(medfilt2(abs(LHRH),[Mh7 Nh7],'symmetric'),2);
[cc,nL]=max(LHRHS(1:round(length(LHRHS)/2)));
[cc,nR]=max(LHRHS(round(length(LHRHS)/2)+1:end));
nR=nR+round(length(LHRHS)/2)+1;
nL(nL>size(LHRH,1))=size(LHRH,1);
nR(nR>size(LHRH,1))=size(LHRH,1);
w5=max(LHRH(nL,:))-min(LHRH(nL,:)); w(5)=w5;
w6=max(LHRH(nR,:))-min(LHRH(nR,:)); w(6)=w6;
[w7,fi]=max(LFFTHRH(nL,6:end));w(7)=w7;
w8=f(fi+5); w(8)=w8;
[w9,fi]=max(LFFTHRH(nR,6:end)); w(9)=w9;
w10=f(fi+5); w(10)=w10;
[cmm,maa]=max(LHRW,[],1);
[w13,w12]=max(cmm); w(13)=w13; w(12)=w12;
w11=maa(w12); w(11)=w11;
if 2*(w(11)-1)>size(LHRW,1)
    LHRW_=LHRW(end:-1:(w(11)-1),:);
    LDHRW=LHRW((w(11)-size(LHRW_,1)+1):w(11),:)-LHRW_;
else
    LDHRW=LHRW(1:w(11),:)-LHRW(2*(w(11)-1):-1:(w(11)-1),:);
end
    w(20)= max(LDHRW(:))-min(LDHRW(:));

h5=ones(19);
LHOW=imresize(conv2(LHO,h5,'valid')/sum(h5(:)),size(LHO));
w(2)=max(max(LHOW));
w(3)=max(LHOW(1,:))-max(LHOW(end,:));
w(4)=max(max(LHOW))-min(min(LHOW));
LHOH=LHO-LHOW;
w=round(w*100)/100;
```

The presented source code is a combination, in the form of a single function, of algorithm fragments provided in the chapters of this monograph (in the area of main image processing and calculating features w. The last stage of this function (*CorvisCalcMain*) is rounding up the values of features w to two decimal places.

The other m-files that were not discussed in full detail are harmonisation of the algorithm portions presented in the previous chapters.

The proposed application has several areas that are deliberately left for attentive readers who would like to independently modify and improve the existing application. In particular, the application does not have:

- any security in the case of exceeding the dimensions of the matrix or in cases where the analyzed matrix is empty (in particular, the calculation performed in the *CorvisCalcMain.m* file),
- the possibility of automated analysis of the patients' folder containing a few tens of patients,
- the possibility of recording information on the time of analysis,
- automatic modification of data of 2D and 3D images and feature values when modifying any of the parameters—it is necessary to press the *ReCalc* button,
- properly adopted data values for functions *polyfit* and *polyval* (*Corvis_Method* file—*Method2*—Fig. 4.35), i.e.: *Warning: Polynomial is badly conditioned. Add points with distinct X values, reduce the degree of the polynomial, or try centering and scaling as described in HELP POLYFIT.*

At this point, I encourage readers to independently improve and supplement the existing application with new elements.

References

1. Shin, J., Lee, J.W., Kim, E.A., Caprioli, J.: The effect of corneal biomechanical properties on rebound tonometer in patients with normal tension glaucoma. Am. J. Ophthalmol. S0002-9394 (14), 00655-2 (2014)
2. Strejc, V.: Naherungsverfahren für aperiodische Übertragungs - charakteristiken. Regelungstechnik 1959, H 4
3. Śródka, W.: Evaluating the material parameters of the human cornea in a numerical model. Acta Bioeng. Biomech. **13**(3), 77–85 (2011)
4. Tian, L., Huang, Y.F., Wang, L.Q., Bai, H., Wang, Q., Jiang, J.J., Wu, Y., Gao, M.: Corneal biomechanical assessment using corneal visualization scheimpflug technology in keratoconic and normal eyes. J. Ophthalmol. **2014**, 147516 (2014)
5. Tian, L., Ko, M.W., Wang, L.K., Zhang, J.Y., Li, T.J., Huang, Y.F., Zheng, Y.P.: Assessment of ocular biomechanics using dynamic ultra high-speed Scheimpflug imaging in keratoconic and normal eyes. J. Refract. Surg. **30**(11), 785–791 (2014)

Chapter 5
Impact of Image Acquisition and Selection of Algorithm Parameters on the Results

The impact of image acquisition, noise in the images and the selection of the algorithm parameters is rarely presented in the literature. This is due to the fact that the authors are afraid that the results obtained will not be in favour of their algorithm or will automatically show its shortcomings and weaknesses. Only in few cases, analysis of this type (the influence of parameters on the results obtained) produces beneficial results which are in favour of the proposed algorithm. This is due to many factors, in particular, testing the algorithm on a small group of images (patient), adoption of a non-representative group of images (for example coming from only one medical centre) or over-matching of the algorithm to data (over-learning). In every algorithm, it is convenient to assume a constant (whatever it is, it does not matter) fitted to the data than calculate it fully automatically. In addition, laboratory (sterile, clean, free from the impact of additional interference) approach to image acquisition does not fully reflect reality. In fact, the measuring path, especially the optical path in the case of a tonometer, is often dirty. The consequence are small artefacts visible in the image and noise. They affect the algorithm operation in a variety of ways. Two main influences can be listed here: measurement error—e.g. of the features from $w(1)$ to $w(20)$, or the error resulting from the incompatibility of the matrix dimensions, e.g. empty matrices which were not created by the algorithm correctly for various reasons.

The methods of image analysis and processing proposed in the previous chapters as well as any methods are sensitive to changing parameters. These parameters are usually: image acquisition methodology and the features, thresholds, adopted in the algorithm. The image acquisition method in the considered tonometer is virtually independent of the operator. However, Gaussian noise or salt and pepper noise may enter the measuring path and be saved in the sequence of recorded images. Equally significant are the adopted values of thresholds p_r described in the previous chapters. A significant number of them are selected fully automatically. However, it is interesting to what extent they affect the obtained results. These issues are discussed thoroughly in the next subchapters.

© Springer International Publishing Switzerland 2016   109
R. Koprowski, *Image Analysis for Ophthalmological Diagnosis*,
Studies in Computational Intelligence 631, DOI 10.1007/978-3-319-29546-6_5

5.1   Impact of Image Acquisition on the Results

The impact of image acquisition on the results obtained can be performed in a number of possible ways. The basic methods, from among those listed above, involve adding noise to the sequence of input images. Among the different types of possible interferences, salt and pepper noise and Gaussian noise were chosen. However, the subject of evaluation is the selected group of features—$w(5)$ and w (13). They were selected due to easy interpretation and a relatively simple relationship with noise. The *imnoise* function with two parameters was used for this purpose:

- 'salt and pepper'—noise density (ns) changed in the range from 0 to 0.5 every 0.01 and
- 'gaussian'—white noise with the mean value equal to zero and variance v changed in the range from 0 to 0.5.

The error δ_w in determining the feature w was measured in the following way:

$$\delta_w = \frac{w_m - w_p}{w_p} \cdot 100\,\% \qquad\qquad (5.1)$$

where:
w_m the measured feature value,
w_p the reference feature value calculated for the corneal image containing no noise.

The results shown in Fig. 5.1 were obtained for the first type of noise (salt and pepper).

The presented results show that the individual feature measurement errors can vary within wide limits. The maximum values of errors are shown in Table 5.1.

The table shows that salt and pepper noise has the least impact on features $w(8)$ and from $w(10)$ to $w(13)$, whereas the largest on features from $w(5)$ to $w(7)$ and w (9). These differences arise from the measurement idea outlined in the previous chapters and thus their varying sensitivity to noise. Attention should be also paid to the degree of noise in images in Fig. 5.1d for $ns = 0.01$, $ns = 0.1$ and $ns = 0.48$ and the correlation with the error values shown in the graph in Fig. 5.1a. The graph in Fig. 5.1a can be divided into two specific areas: an increase in the value of error δ_w for $ns \in (0, 0.025]$ and its decrease for $ns \in (0.025, 0.5)$. Seemingly, a higher noise value results in a smaller feature measurement error. However, only the feature values are taken into account and there is no interpretation of the accuracy of the data on whose basis they are calculated. For example, Fig. 5.2 shows changes in the contour shape of the image L_H that forms the basis for the calculation of the features w for $ns \in \{0, 0.001, 0.003, 0.005, 0.01, 0.02, 0.05, 0.1\}$.

Therefore, changes in the error value for ns below 0.02 are not meaningful.

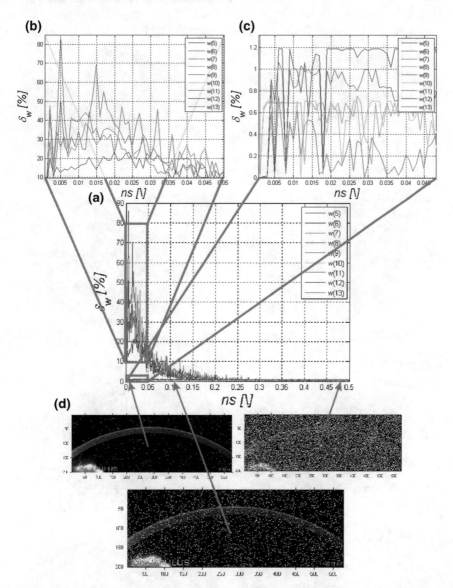

Fig. 5.1 Graph of the error δ_w of the features from $w(5)$ to $w(13)$ as a function of noise density (salt and pepper) (**a**); enlarged portions of the graph **b–d** sample images of the cornea for $ns = 0.01$, $ns = 0.1$ and $ns = 0.48$ respectively

Table 5.1 Summary of the maximum measurement errors of the features from $w(5)$ to $w(13)$

Feature	$w(5)$	$w(6)$	$w(7)$	$w(8)$	$w(9)$	$w(10)$	$w(11)$	$w(12)$	$w(13)$
max δ_w	23	50	47	0.8	86	0.7	1.1	1.2	1

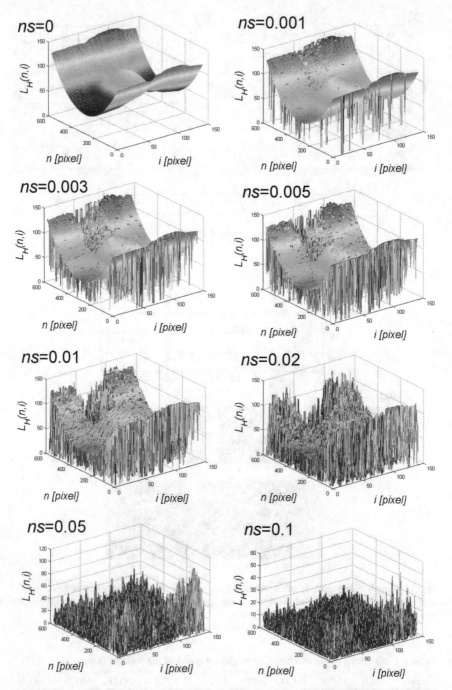

Fig. 5.2 Changes in the shape of the image L_H for $ns \in \{0, 0.001, 0.003, 0.005, 0.01, 0.02, 0.05, 0.1\}$

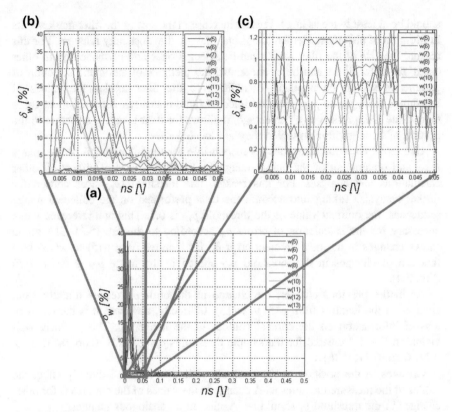

Fig. 5.3 Graph of the error δ_w of the features from $w(5)$ to $w(13)$ in the variance function v (Gaussian) (**a**); enlarged portions of the graph **b–d** sample images of the cornea for, $v = 0.01$, $v = 0.1$ and $v = 0.48$ respectively

The changes in the error δ_w of features from $w(5)$ to $w(13)$ for Gaussian noise look similar. The results are shown in Fig. 5.3.

Compared to salt and pepper noise, feature measurement errors δ_w are smaller in the case of Gaussian noise. For example, for $w(9)$ the maximum error is 38 %, whereas in the case of salt and pepper noise its value reached 86 % (see Table 5.1). The features from $w(5)$ to $w(13)$ have varying degrees of sensitivity to both the type of noise and its various values. I encourage readers to perform a similar analysis for the other features.

5.2 Impact of the Selection of the Algorithm Parameters on the Results

In this monograph several parameters, selected in different ways, were used. The sizes of filter masks and structural elements resulted mainly from the size and type of interference. When the size of interference is known, the filter mask (e.g. median)

should be at least twice as large. Further increase in the size of the filter mask results in filtration of also these elements, objects, that are diagnostically relevant. For this reason, the size of the filter masks can be selected once and permanently. In other cases, for other filters and other situations, the methods of automatic selection of parameters should be applied. In addition to the filter masks, the values of thresholds from p_{r1} to p_{r13} are also selected (automatically). Since in most cases their value is expressed as a percentage, it allows for their adaptive selection to the portion of the algorithm in which they are located.

One example is the threshold p_{r7} responsible for the binarization of the image L_{GAS} and obtainment of the output image L_H being the basis of almost all other calculations and analyses. For this reason, this threshold (p_{r7}) was chosen for further analysis. Taking into account the tests performed on the collected image sequences, the optimal value of the threshold p_{r7} is 0.1. This is a reference value necessary for the calculation of errors δ_w according to the Eq. (5.1). The graph shows changes in the measurement error δ_w for features from $w(5)$ to $w(13)$ as a function of changes in the threshold p_{r7} altered in the range $p_{r7} \in (0.01, 0.5)$ (Fig. 5.4).

As in the previous chapter, the change in the error δ_w results directly from changes in the features from $w(5)$ to $w(13)$. Indirectly, however, it is the result of loss of information on the corneal contour in the image L_H. This is fairly well visible in Fig. 5.5 created for the sample thresholds $p_{r7} \in \{0.01, 0.06, 0.11, 0.16, 0.21, 0.26, 0.31, 0.36\}$.

Changes in the position of the contours visible in Fig. 5.5 directly affect the values of the measured features w. A change in the values of the features w for other changes in the threshold p_r should be verified in an analogous manner.

Taking into account the obtained results, the area of analysis of the signal-to-noise (S/N) ratio for the image L_H when changing parameters remains open (please see Figs. 5.2 and 5.5). It is also possible to conduct additional studies

Fig. 5.4 Graph showing the relationship between the error δ_w and the threshold $p_{r7} \in$ (0.01, 0.5) when $p_{r7} = 0.1$ is assumed as the reference value (**a**); enlarged portions of the graph (**b**) and (**c**)

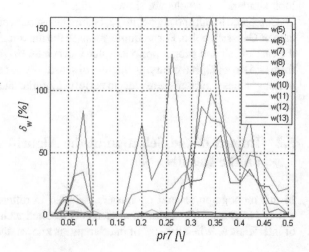

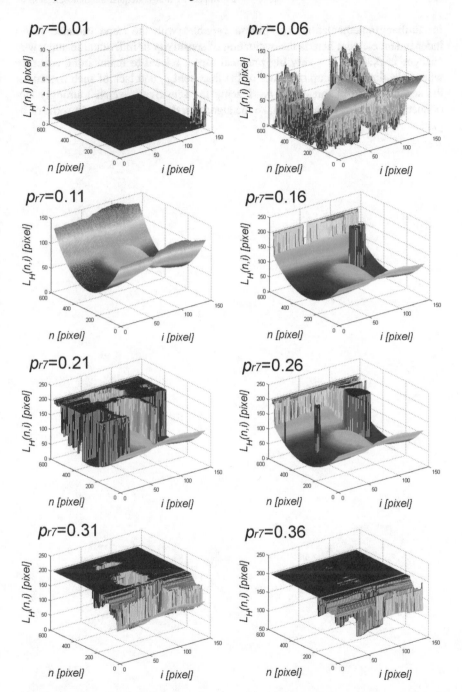

Fig. 5.5 Changes in the shape of the image L_H for $p_{r7} \in \{0.01, 0.06, 0.11, 0.16, 0.21, 0.26, 0.31, 0.36\}$

for further implementations of random variables with the same variance v. An independent element here is the evaluation of sensitivity of individual features w to changes in p_r. This is a very big practical aspect related to maintaining accuracy when selecting one group of values of the threshold p_r and lack of such a need for the second group of thresholds p_r. Tracing the sensitivity, which I strongly recommend the reader, enables to make the algorithm designer sensitive to some of its parts.

Chapter 6
Summary of Measured Features

Below there is a summary of the measured features described in the chapters of this monograph (Table 6.1).

Table 6.1 Summary of features measured in the proposed application and described in this monograph

Feature	Object	Description
$w(1)$	Eyeball + cornea	Contrast calculated on the basis of the GLCM analysis of the corneal texture
$w(2)$	Eyeball	Maximum amplitude of the high harmonic of the eyeball reaction
$w(3)$	Eyeball	Difference between the maximum values of the eyeball reaction for low frequencies calculated for the extreme positions in the n axis
$w(4)$	Eyeball	Difference between the maximum values of the eyeball reaction for high frequencies calculated for the full range of data
$w(5)$	Eyeball	Maximum difference between the minimum and maximum amplitude for each i at the point n_L
$w(6)$	Eyeball	Maximum difference between the minimum and maximum amplitude for each i at the point n_R
$w(7)$	Eyeball	Value of the maximum amplitude in the spectrum of the eyeball reaction for $f \in (100, 490)$ Hz at the point n_L
$w(8)$	Eyeball	Frequency value for the maximum amplitude in the spectrum of the eyeball reaction for $f \in (100, 490)$ Hz at the point n_L
$w(9)$	Eyeball	Value of the maximum amplitude in the spectrum of the eyeball reaction for $f \in (100, 490)$ Hz at the point n_R
$w(10)$	Eyeball	Frequency value for the maximum amplitude in the spectrum of the eyeball reaction for $f \in (100, 490)$ Hz at the point n_R
$w(11)$	Cornea	Location in the column axis of the maximum amplitude of a low-frequency corneal response to force
$w(12)$	Cornea	Location in the i axis of the maximum amplitude of a low-frequency corneal response to force
$w(13)$	Cornea	Value of the maximum amplitude of a low-frequency corneal response to force

(continued)

© Springer International Publishing Switzerland 2016
R. Koprowski, *Image Analysis for Ophthalmological Diagnosis*,
Studies in Computational Intelligence 631, DOI 10.1007/978-3-319-29546-6_6

Table 6.1 (continued)

Feature	Object	Description
$w(14)$	Cornea	Location of the first applanation in the i axis
$w(15)$	Cornea	Location of the second applanation in the i axis
$w(16)$	Cornea	Notional value of the corneal deformation amplitude for the first applanation
$w(17)$	Cornea	Notional value of the corneal deformation amplitude for the second applanation
$w(18)$	Cornea	Time constant $Tz - Tm$—the rate of the corneal response to force
$w(19)$	Cornea	Time constant Tz—transport delay of the corneal response to force
$w(20)$	Cornea	Difference in the corneal response between the left and right side calculated from the maximum deformation

Individual features can be also easily found in subsequent parts of the algorithm provided in the monograph and attached m-files. The nomenclature is only slightly modified in the source code. The symbols of individual features have been changed from the number of position in the matrix w to the symbol with a number, for example, the feature $w(12)$ has a symbol $w12$ in the source code and so on.

Chapter 7
Conclusions

Methods for analysis of corneal deformation images from the Corvis tonometer can be different. This monograph shows only one of the possible approaches to image analysis and one of possible GUI solutions. The presented solution works well in medical practice providing a number of additional parameters impossible to obtain in the Corvis tonometer software. Their interpretation and finding the link with the type of the patient's disease constitute the next step of analysis. Surely it should be the analysis made using one of classification possibilities (e.g. available in Matlab): decision trees, neural networks, naive Bayesian classifier or support vector machine (SVM). For this purpose there are profiled functions/toolboxes: *classregtree*, *Neural Network Toolbox*, *predict*, *svmtrain* and *svmclassify* respectively. They should be used to verify if classification is correct for the data coming from different medical institutions. The number of features used for classification should also be limited to the most significant ones and at least three times smaller than the number of analysed cases. Classification results, at the stage of training the classifier, should be verified by an ophthalmologist (expert) or compared with other measurement results obtained using more accurate methods. This will prevent excessive over-fitting to the data, which is also the consequence of excessive algorithmic profiling [1]. The classification of patients may therefore relate to various diseases and issues: for example, the impact of keratoconus, IOP, Age-related Macular Degeneration (AMD) or diabetes to changes in features w. Thus the features w, whose measurement method is presented in this monograph, can be used in many different ways. In extreme cases, the proposed algorithm can be also profiled for use in other fields of ophthalmology and medicine. The GUI can be modified in any way by choosing other parameters associated with the location of buttons and images. The given source code also enables to compile and use modules of the algorithm in C language. It is therefore possible to combine fragments of the presented algorithm with the existing Corvis tonometer software. Finally, the presented algorithms and this monograph, due to the full availability of source codes without any limitation, can be used for teaching purposes, as one example of using Matlab in teaching. In conclusion, I would like to encourage readers to make their own modifications and improvements in the presented application. Perhaps this approach will increase the popularity and versatility of measurements and diagnostics using the Corvis tonometer.

© Springer International Publishing Switzerland 2016
R. Koprowski, *Image Analysis for Ophthalmological Diagnosis*,
Studies in Computational Intelligence 631, DOI 10.1007/978-3-319-29546-6_7

Reference

1. Foster, K.R., Koprowski, R., Skufca, J.D.: Machine learning, medical diagnosis, and biomedical engineering research—commentary. Biomed. Eng. Online **13**, 94 (2014)

Appendix

In order to facilitate testing of the algorithms presented in this monograph, m-files are also available in the form of additional files. These files are compressed (zipped) in three containers:

- *pre_processing.zip*—contains three m-files which enable to create the GUI related to image pre-processing:

  - *Corvis_GUI.m*—graphical user interface,
  - *CorvisCalcPre.m*—calculations relating to image pre-processing,
  - *CorvisFunction.m*—functions called from the GUI.

- *processing.zip*—contains six m-files which enable to create the GUI related to pre-processing and main processing of images (Note—files: *CorvisGUI.m, CorvisCalcPre.m and CorvisFunction.m* differ in comparison with the files from the *pre_processing.zip* container):

  - *CorvisGUI.m*—responsible for placement of buttons, images, and other menu items,
  - *CorvisFunction.m*—responsible for the type and form of response to pressing a button or another action of the user,
  - *CorvisCalcPre.m*—image pre-processing function,
  - *CorvisCalcMain.m*—function intended for main image processing,
  - *Corvis_Method.m*—function designed to select the desired main processing method (discussed in Chapter 3 Main image processing),
  - *CorvisExcel_write.m*—function designed to write selected results to an Excel file.

- *book.zip*—contains 33 m-files directly related to individual chapters of this monograph. The name of each m-file correlates with the number of chapters. The names contain a shortcut which suggests their purpose. In the order of chapters, these are:

  - *Chapter_1_detect_contour1.m*
  - *Chapter_1_detect_contour2.m*
  - *Chapter_1_detect_contour3.m*

© Springer International Publishing Switzerland 2016
R. Koprowski, *Image Analysis for Ophthalmological Diagnosis*,
Studies in Computational Intelligence 631, DOI 10.1007/978-3-319-29546-6

- *Chapter_2_read_data.m*
- *Chapter_2_read_data.m*
- *Chapter_2_read_data2.m*
- *Chapter_2_imnoise.m*
- *Chapter_2_normalization.m*
- *Chapter_2_background.m*
- *Chapter_2_background2.m*
- *Chapter_2_image_hist_equ.m*
- *Chapter_3_edge_detector.m*
- *Chapter_3_edge_detector2.m*
- *Chapter_3_filter_hist.m*
- *Chapter_3_contour_label_filter.m*
- *Chapter_3_contour_LF.m*
- *Chapter_3_contour_LH.m*
- *Chapter_3_contour_LH2.m*
- *Chapter_3_contour_LE.m*
- *Chapter_3_comparison_new_methods.m*
- *Chapter_3_contour_LE_filter*
- *Chapter_4_texture.m*
- *Chapter_4_texture_2.m*
- *Chapter_4_eye_left_right.m*
- *Chapter_4_frequency_analysis.m*
- *Chapter_4_frequency_analysis2.m*
- *Chapter_4_cornea_applanation.m*
- *Chapter_4_cornea_reconstruct_3D.m*
- *Chapter_4_cornea_symmetry.m*
- *Chapter_5_influence_noise.m*
- *Chapter_5_influence_noise_2.m*
- *Chapter_5_influence_noise_3.m*
- *Chapter_5_influence_pr_3D.m*
- *Chapter_5_influence_pr_2_3D.m*
- *Chapter_5_influence_pr_3D.m*

All files are part and parcel of this book. However, if they have not been provided with it, they are also available for download from http://extras.springer. com.

Advertising

Measuring Biomechanical Properties in Vivo
The Corvis® ST

Measuring biomechanical properties is currently one of the most challenging fields in modern ophthalmology. Until now it was not possible to measure the elastic or viscous properties of the cornea in vivo. However, the possible applications would be numerous since several diseases such as keratoconus have their origin in the change of corneal biomechanical properties. Not surprisingly, during the recent years the interest has arisen to predict corneal response to corneal treatment or to disease related changes in corneal properties.

Ultra High-Speed Scheimpflug Camera in Combination with Air-Pulse Tonometry

Scheimpflug imaging offers the advantage of a very high temporal and spatial resolution at the same time and a higher depth of focus compared to conventional slit imaging techniques.

The Corvis® ST (Corneal Visualization Scheimpflug Technology) is the first commercially available high-speed imaging device in combination with a Gaussian shaped air-pulse. The ultra-high speed Scheimpflug camera captures 4,430 frames

© Springer International Publishing Switzerland 2016   123
R. Koprowski, *Image Analysis for Ophthalmological Diagnosis*,
Studies in Computational Intelligence 631, DOI 10.1007/978-3-319-29546-6

per second. Immediately before the air pulse starts the anterior segment of the eye is illuminated by blue light through a 9 mm slit. Based on the Scheimpflug images before the deformation of the cornea has started the system can also measure corneal thickness. In the 31 ms after the beginning of the air pulse the high-speed camera captures 140 frames of the illuminated horizontal sectional plane.

The 140 images that are captured while the air pulse is applied, depict a clear image of the deformation process. The recording starts with the cornea in the initial state. The beginning air pulse forces the cornea inwards through applanation into a concavity phase until it achieves the highest concavity. Before the cornea returns into its original state, a second applanation moment occurs. Figure shows a series of images during the deformation of the cornea as a response to the air pulse.

Evaluation of the Dynamic Corneal Response (DCR) with the Corvis® ST

During the complete deformation several parameters describe the specific response of the measured cornea to the defined air pulse. This versatile information extracted from the direct view of the corneal deformation results in clinically relevant parameters correlated with biomechanical properties.

One important parameter that is strongly dependent on biomechanical properties is the Radius of Curvature during deformation. The Radius of curvature describes the curvature of the central part of the cornea in the concave phase of the deformation. Recent studies have shown that this parameter is highly correlated with biomechanical change such as stiffness changes after corneal crosslinking or after refractive laser surgery, whereas changes of intraocular pressure have only minor contributions to changes of this parameter.

In conclusion, the combination of a high-speed Scheimpflug camera with an air-pulse tonometer provides a detailed view of the biomechanical response of the cornea. Several Corvis ST parameters generated by the Corvis ST® provide a clinical in vivo characterization of corneal biomechanical properties, which is relevant for different applications in ophthalmology.

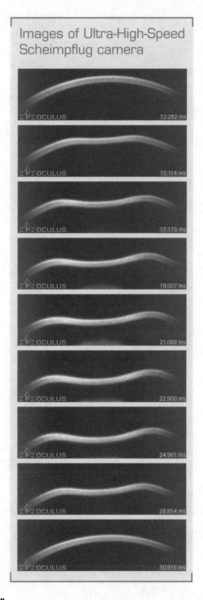

Dr. Sven Reisdorf